SOTHIS PRESS

Sothis Press aims to completely reimagine the public domain book with an emphasis on universal access to captivatingly designed print editions. We believe that technology will enable every single book ever published to be perpetually accessible in beautiful print form. Sothis is beauty in ubiquity.

www.sothis.press
1 Waterhouse Square, London, ECIN 2ST

Before the Doctor Comes

A Ready Reference Book, Giving the Symptoms of Common Diseases, and Indicating Proper Emergency Treatment in Case of Sudden Illness or Accident Pending the Physician's Arrival

Mary M. Crawford

SOTHIS PRESS

ISBN 978-1-0365-2524-8

Before the Doctor Comes
is in the public domain.

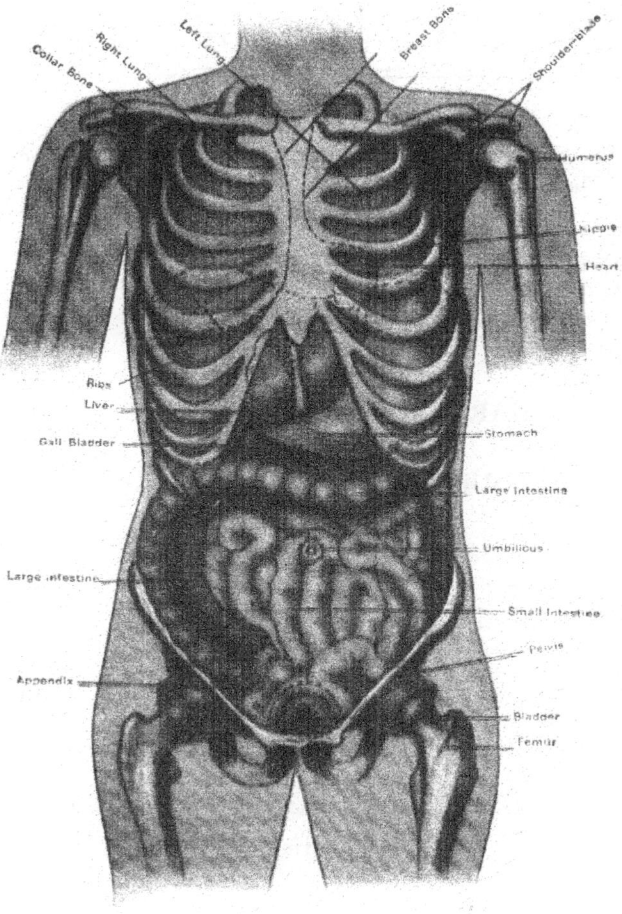

INTERNAL ORGANS OF THE BODY

Before the Doctor Comes

A Ready Reference Book, Giving the Symptoms of Common Diseases, and Indicating Proper Emergency Treatment in Case of Sudden Illness or Accident Pending the Physician's Arrival

BY

MARY M. CRAWFORD, M.D.,

AND

THURSTON S. WELTON, M.D.

NEW YORK
THE CHRISTIAN HERALD
LOUIS KLOPSCH, PROPRIETOR
BIBLE HOUSE

The Purpose of This Book

Most people have an imperfect knowledge of medical matters. Their ideas of disease and sickness are derived from tradition, from advertisements, and from so-called medical information received from all sorts of ignorant persons. In an emergency the chances are that the ordinary individual will do the wrong thing.

In the experience of physicians it is known that, in many cases, a doctor is called in to see a patient when it is too late to be of much service. The friends and relatives thought they recognized some common ailment that would pass away of itself, and after the disease had wrecked the life of the patient, the doctor was called. This happens every day. Very often, too, a physician is hurriedly sent for when a little knowledge and simple practical remedies would clear up the mystery and save the expense of medical advice.

What to do before the doctor comes and when to call him in, are what this book aims to teach.

Its purpose is not to make ready-made doctors, but to enlighten, to give the proper view-point, to instruct in the first laws of health, to teach what to do in an emergency, and to explain the gravity of certain conditions and symptoms that need the skill of a competent physician.

The authors' intention is to speak plainly—technical terms are only used when absolutely necessary; scientific discussions or descriptions are put in readable words—and every effort has been made to enable the reader to understand every word. While to a physician this book is but a primer, it has been written along strictly ethical lines. No new theories have been advanced, no special drugs have been recommended and no new cult or teaching has been explained.

It may happen, when one in the family is sick, that a nurse is needed. Perhaps it is beyond the means of the family to employ one, or perhaps, especially in the country, none can be procured. Therefore, the family has to do the nursing. Nursing is an art in itself, and this book cannot, in a few pages, make skilful nurses. But there are points of nursing that have been fully described. The care of the sick, the keeping of the sick-room, the proper way to make a sick-bed, the proper method of recording the pulse, temperature and respiration of the patient, the proper food for the sick, according to the disease, the preparation of different dishes, the method of giving medicine, the making of poultices, the giving of enemas or rectal injections, and numerous other points have been fully described. These are things that every intelligent person should know. It is the aim of this book to make all these things clear.

The first chapter is devoted to a general description of the human body, without knowledge of which the remaining chapters could not be intelligently studied.

We hope that those who read this book carefully will be repaid for the effort. Many things will be learned not known before, and the reader will be better able to do the right thing at the right time, before the doctor comes.

MARY M. CRAWFORD, M. D.
THURSTON S. WELTON, M. D.

Brooklyn, 1909.

CONTENTS

CHAPTER I

The Normal Body

CHAPTER II

Hygiene

CHAPTER III

First Aid

CONTENTS

PAGE

CHAPTER VII

Diseases of the Nervous System

CHAPTER VIII

Diseases of the Eye, Ear, Nose and Throat

CHAPTER IX

General Diseases

PAGE

CHAPTER X

Diseases of the Blood and Heart

CHAPTER XI

Diseases of the Kidney and Bladder

CHAPTER XII

Infectious and Contagious Diseases

CHAPTER XIII

Diseases of Children

CHAPTER XIV

Surgical Conditions

CHAPTER XV

Care of the Infant

CHAPTER XVI

Home Nursing

ILLUSTRATIONS

ILLUSTRATIONS

Before the Doctor Comes

CHAPTER I

THE NORMAL BODY

The human body is made up of different structures and organs. Each of these has its own function; yet no one is independent of any other, and the body needs them all, working harmoniously and efficiently, to maintain itself in a normal, healthy state.

If the human body be regarded as a building, it may be said to have a foundation, framework and superstructure. The details of the building are the Bones, Muscles, Nerves, Fat and an outside covering, the Skin, which encloses the various organs of the body. There are three main cavities of the body, the cranial or head cavity, the thoracic or chest cavity, and the abdominal cavity below the chest. Other cavities are the eye, ear and nose cavities and the mouth.

The Skeleton may be called the framework and perhaps foundation of the structure. It consists of 206 bones, united together by various devices of nature so as to permit of the numerous motions of the body. These bones differ in size and shape. There are long bones, flat bones, round bones and irregularly shaped bones. The long bones are those of the legs and arms, fingers and toes; the round bones are the small bones of the wrist and ankle and the knee cap; the flat bones form the head, the breast bone and the ribs; the vertebræ, or elements of the spinal column, and some of the head bones comprise the irregularly shaped bones. The bones are joined to each other by joints, some permitting liberal movement, as at the shoulder, and others permitting only limited motion, as at the articulation of the ribs and the spinal column. The bones at the joints are lined with a smooth membrane, which secretes an oily fluid which lubricates the joint, thus facilitating free motion. Outside of this membrane are the ligaments, or tough bands, which keep the bone-ends forming the joint in proper position. Muscles are attached to both bones, by which the joint is operated.

The vertebral column or spine is the mainstay of the human body. The head rests upon and is upheld by it. The ribs are attached to it, and its hollow interior forms a tube which contains the spinal cord and has numerous openings from which the nerves emerge. Made up of bones separated by elastic cartilage, it can bend in any direction and by this means mitigate any shock transmitted from other parts of the body.

Muscles.—The muscles enable the body to move; they are of two kinds, voluntary and involuntary. The involuntary muscles are those of breathing, the heart muscle, and the muscles of the stomach and intestine. These muscles do their work constantly and without any exercise of the will. Other muscles are under control of the will and can be used or not at pleasure. In fact, the will must act or these muscles will not act. This act of the will may be so rapid as to be automatic, as, for instance, the mental operation involved in playing the piano. Take, again, the case of a person who thoughtlessly touches a hot surface. He feels the burn, the impression flashes to the brain, and the brain signals to remove the finger, all before the muscle can act; but the finger is withdrawn without consciousness of this double mental operation. All this is accomplished by means of the nerves.

Nerves.—These are long fine threads of soft tissue reaching from the brain and spinal cord to every part of the body, but especially the surface. Along these threads intelligence is transmitted more quickly than on telegraph wires.

Nerves are either motor or sensory. The former transmit to the muscles orders sent by the brain; the latter transmit sensations from the surface of the body to the brain. If a motor nerve is cut, all the muscles controlled by that nerve cease to move; if a sensory nerve is cut, so much of the surface of the body as uses that nerve, loses the sense of feeling. When a person is paralyzed, the cause is usually a break in the natural connection between brain and motor nerves, generally caused by pressure of a clot of blood.

There is a third system of nerves, constituting the sympathetic system, which are connected with internal organs, enabling them to perform their functions properly.

Fat.—Fat is deposited in various parts of the body. Even thin people have some. It is really food and fuel for the body. In prolonged sickness and in case of starvation, the body consumes its own fat, which also supplies the body with heat in the process of being used up. With some persons, fat-production becomes a disease; the body seems unable to stop it, and they attain immense size, which no exercising or dieting can reduce. People who live in cold climates usually have more fat than those in temperate zones, for the food necessary in a cold climate has more fat and oils in it; and nature also tends to give such people more fat as a natural protection against the cold.

Skin.—Most people look upon the skin merely as a covering of the body. But it is far more than that; it is an organ of the body and a very complex one. Throughout the skin there are minute glands, called the sweat glands, from which are excreted all sorts of waste products of the body. We cannot live unless these glands perform their function properly. If even three-fourths of the skin of a man were varnished over so that these glands could not excrete, he would die. Hence, to keep the skin in healthy condition is very important for the general health of the body. There are other glands in the skin, called sebaceous glands, which secrete an oily substance which keeps the skin soft and prevents it from drying up and cracking.

In the skin, too, are situated all the delicate sensory nerve-endings which tell us when it is cold or hot, when things are soft or hard. This function is a great protection to us, for without such instantaneous and delicate perception, our bodies might be burnt, frozen, bruised and destroyed before we became aware of any trouble.

Brain and Spinal Cord.—The brain and spinal cord constitute what is known as the Central Nervous System.

Two kinds of tissue make up the brain and cord: the gray and the white. The "gray matter" of the brain is the tissue in which thought is supposed to originate. The white matter is the connecting substance which holds the gray matter in place. The brain has various centres in its surface which control different functions of the body. The relation between some parts of the brain and certain functions of the body is well known, but many such relations remain still undiscovered. The brain centres which control the arms, legs, face, etc., have been identified; but this part of medical science is in its infancy.

Certain nerves lead directly from the brain to the head and face, such as nerves of hearing, sight, taste and smell. Other nerves pass from the brain down the spinal cord, and then emerge through openings in the spinal column to reach different parts of the body.

By means of the brain and spinal cord the body performs its functions. Without these, human life, as we know it, would be impossible. Nervous exhaustion, implying as it does the enfeebling of the brain and nervous system, is a very serious matter.

Digestive System.—This includes the whole digestive apparatus, from the mouth to the rectum, and is in effect a hollow tube or channel, continuous from one end to the other. From the mouth food passes into the œsophagus, a muscular tube leading to the stomach. The stomach is an expansion of the tube, holding from a pint to a quart, but capable of dilatation beyond this measure. In the stomach, the food is made to move about by muscular contractions of the walls of the stomach. From the stomach the partly digested food passes into the upper part of the small intestine, called the duodenum. Here the process of digestion continues and the food advances through other parts of the small intestine, which is about twenty-three feet long and is coiled up in the abdominal cavity. It is directly connected with the large intestine, and at the point of connection the appendix is found. This is a small tube closed at one end, about as long as the little finger and not so thick, with a narrow bore. Inflammation of this organ is called appendicitis. The large intestine begins in the lower right side of the abdomen, and after several turns it enters the pelvic cavity and is there called the rectum. Through the rectum occurs the daily bowel movement, when the body rejects the waste products of digestion and that food which it cannot use. Waste material retained in the intestines becomes real poison, which may be absorbed so as to find its way into the circulation, whence it attacks the nervous system. Hence constipation must be avoided. Children should be taught that a daily movement of the bowels is as important as it is to eat.

Lungs.—The lungs are the essential organs of breathing. There are two lungs, one right and one left. The lungs contain innumerable tiny cells, which receive fresh air and expel exhausted air. Upward from the lungs the windpipe or trachea extends to the larynx or voice-box, which any one may feel by pressing the front of the neck. When largely developed, it is called the "Adam's apple." This larynx opens into the throat through the glottis, back of the tongue. Just above the larynx a piece of cartilage, or tough elastic tissue, called the epiglottis, works on a sort of hinge, opening for the passage of air and closing when food or liquid is swallowed. The diaphragm, a muscular partition, separates the chest from the abdominal cavity. In breathing this contracts and expands, with the chest walls. As the chest cavity becomes larger by this expansion the lungs expand and air rushes in and fills them; as the cavity contracts, exhausted air is expelled. The lining of the air cells of the lungs contains blood vessels, with very thin walls. As fresh air enters the air cells, it is absorbed by the blood, and at the same time certain waste products are released from the blood and become the warm breath (carbon dioxide) which is constantly exhaled. With each breath fresh air is given to the blood for the tissue and the used-up air is cast out. From this it appears that if a man stays for hours in a closed room without fresh air he will soon use up the oxygen, which is the vital element in the air. In such a room the man feels dull, his head aches, and he cannot think. If he remains long enough without fresh air he will die by slow suffocation. In the chapter treating of personal hygiene, we discuss the necessity for fresh air and correct breathing.

The Heart.—The heart is a hollow muscular pump which forces blood to all parts of the body. It is placed in the chest cavity, almost in the middle line, but with the apex extending to the left, so that the heart-beat is felt at the left.

In the circulation of the blood two large veins (*vena cava* ascending and descending), convey the impure blood into the right auricle of the heart, whence it passes into the right ventricle. The right ventricle pumps this blood through valves, which open one way and thus prevent blood once pumped onward from returning, into the arteries which carry the blood to the lungs. Here it comes in contact with the fresh air and the changes already noticed take place. From the lungs the refreshed blood passes to the left auricle of the heart, from which it is pumped into the left ventricle, and thence into the main artery of the body, the *aorta,* and so on all through the body until the capillaries are reached. These vessels are microscopic in size, and it is from them that the tissues receive nourishment from the fresh blood, while at the same time they empty into the blood waste products of the body. This impure blood finds its way through the veins, where it shows a blue color, back into the two large veins leading into the heart.

The muscles of the heart contract (in health) regularly and without any exercise of the will. The number of beats per minute varies. From 72 to 80 times per minute is normal for an adult. A child's rate may be from 100 to 120, or even 140 in the case of babies.

Liver.—The liver, the largest single organ of the body, lies in the right upper part of the abdomen close to the diaphragm. It is more bulky than the heart or the lungs. Immediately below it and attached to its under surface is the gall-bladder, and the duodenum lies close against it. The gall-bladder and liver act together in secreting and storing a fluid called "bile," which has an important function in the process of digestion.

Secreted by the liver, the bile finds its way through the bile ducts, gall-bladder and gall duct into the duodenum, where it assists digestion.

Pancreas.—The pancreas is a long, flat, lobulated organ lying across the body, behind and below the stomach.

It secretes important digestive juices which enter the duodenum through the pancreatic duct. These juices are alkaline in character and not acid as are the digestive juices of the stomach. Starchy food, fats and proteid are digested by the pancreatic fluid.

The Spleen is one of the ductless glands, and is believed to produce an internal secretion taken up directly by the blood. It is found in the left upper part of the abdominal cavity.

The functions of this organ are not thoroughly understood. Spleens have been entirely removed without inconvenience to the patients.

The Thyroid Gland is situated in the neck below the larynx. This gland produces an internal secretion, which has an important relation to the normal development of both mind and body. Some children called cretins, whose condition approximates to idiocy, are born with diseased thyroids. Their physical development is imperfect, the head is large, intelligence is lacking, and later in life there is commonly a large swelling of the gland in the neck, known as goitre. This condition is rare in the United States.

Kidneys and Bladder.—The kidneys lie close to the spine and the last two ribs. Their function is to receive waste matter from the blood and excrete it in the urine which passes from the kidneys into the bladder. The bladder is a hollow, muscular organ, which receives the urine and discharges it by muscular effort.

CHAPTER II

HYGIENE

PERSONAL HYGIENE

Personal hygiene includes the care of all the different organs and functions of the body, so that a state of health may be maintained and the individual may have the full, free use of his powers. Hence, for each person the rules will differ slightly, as each person's strength, character and general physical as well as mental make-up differ from every other person's. In a book like this, only a brief discussion of the subject is possible. For convenience, personal hygiene has been divided into several sub-headings, as follows: breathing, sleeping, bathing, eating, drinking, clothing, exercise, home conditions, etc. These will be taken up in order. The reader must modify these suggestions to suit his particular condition or situation.

Breathing.—There are two important points to be considered in breathing:

1. The manner of breathing.

2. The quality of the air we breathe.

People who work indoors do not realize that they habitually fill only part of the lungs with fresh air. An ordinary breath taken when a person is quiet does not change the air in more than one quarter of the lungs. The air at the base of the lungs and at the apex is not changed except by very deep breathing. This is one reason why people who live and work indoors are more likely than others to contract consumption. Their lungs are not kept healthy and strong by proper exercise and sufficient fresh air; and so, when the germ of consumption is inhaled, the tissue of the lungs is not vigorous enough to destroy it.

Every night and morning, and, indeed, throughout the day, people should exercise their lungs by deep, full inspirations (preferably through the nose) in the open air. Draw in as much as you can and then slowly let it out. Repeat this, not too rapidly, half a dozen times. Naturally, the best way is to do all this unconsciously in the course of vigorous exercise. That will be discussed later; the above is for those who do not or cannot get adequate exercise.

The second factor in correct breathing, *i. e.*, the quality of the air, is also too little considered. Every well person should spend part of each day in the open air and sunshine, and every sick person should have all the fresh air and sunshine that is possible. Nature gives these two gifts free and if we use them rightly there will be less sickness in the world.

At night when we sleep the body is storing up strength and new tissue for the next day's waste. At this time, the blood takes more oxygen from the air to replenish the tissues. Hence, even more important than fresh air in the day is sufficient and continued fresh air at night. Every one, no matter what the season, should sleep with open windows. Be sure to have sufficient covering and even a night-cap, if the head is sensitive; but let the bedroom have a good supply of fresh air all through the night.

Sleeping.—No rule fixing hours of sleep can be laid down for all people. Some can do more work with less sleep than others. But each person has a rule for himself. He discovers that unless he sleeps a certain number of hours he will suffer for it. For some people five or six hours of sleep seem to be enough; others must have eight and some need even twelve. Sleep taken at regular times in regular amounts does more good than irregular sleep. The body when accustomed to a certain routine does its best work. If a night's rest is lost in part, it is better to make it up the next night by sleeping four or five hours longer, than to sleep in the daytime. Invalids and very delicate people need more sleep and need it oftener. Too much sleep is as bad as too little. Lazy habits are formed, fat is induced, dullness and disinclination to work result. If a young person suddenly develops this habit, be sure there is something wrong. Usually it means the intestines are absorbing certain toxins or poisons which they should cast off with the *excreta*. A good cathartic, such as castor oil or the old-fashioned brimstone and molasses, will often be sufficient to correct this trouble.

Bathing.—To be ordinarily clean three baths a week are necessary. This practice will remove the dead scales of the skin, the external secretions of the body, and the outside dirt which accumulates. But to be absolutely clean and at the same time to keep the skin and general condition at their best a daily bath is necessary. This is a luxury which every one cannot enjoy, but those who can should bathe daily, and those who cannot should at least sponge themselves off once a day.

Many people take a cold bath in the morning. This is very fine as a tonic and stimulant for those who are strong enough to react from it. But

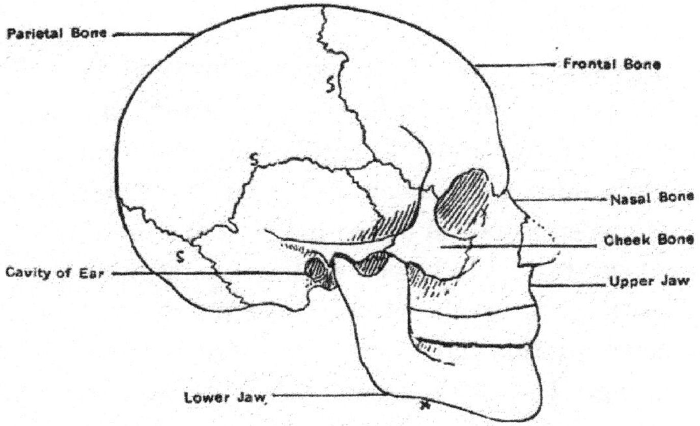

BONES OF SKULL

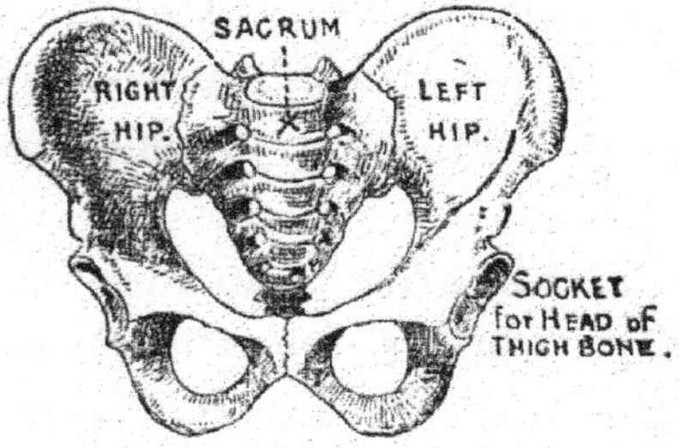

THE PELVIS, MADE UP OF RIGHT AND LEFT HIP BONES AND THE SACRUM

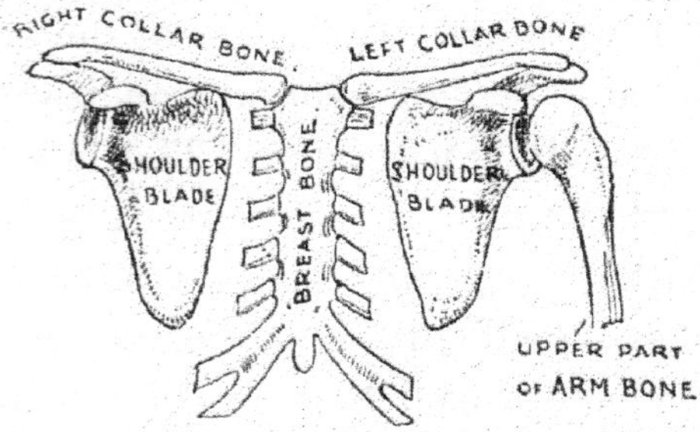

UPPER CHEST, SHOWING THE RELATIONS OF THE SHOULDER-BLADES, THE COLLAR BONES AND THE BREAST BONE

others should not indulge. If after a cold bath the bather feels a healthy glow, if the skin becomes pink after the rub-down, and if he feels stronger and better, the bath is good for him and should be continued. But if there is no after-glow, if the lips become blue or pale, if the bather feels tired or exhausted, he should not think of continuing the practice. Instead, a tepid bath should be substituted.

During the summer, sea bathing or fresh-water bathing cannot be too highly recommended, along with the healthy exercise of swimming. People should not stay in the water too long or they will feel exhausted and chilled and may contract severe colds. About half an hour is a safe limit. Mothers should remember that small children lose their body heat faster than an adult. Hence, a child of five or six should not stay in the water as long as an older person.

After eating, bathing should not be undertaken for a considerable space of time. Two or three hours is a safe limit. Severe cramps have been known to attack persons entering cold water too soon after a hearty meal. Do not enter the cold sea water while heated from violent exercise, but wait until moderately cooled off. Upon first entering the water, be sure to wet the head. This may prevent headache, and, in very hot weather, even sun-stroke.

A Tepid Bath is one from 80° to 90° Fahrenheit. It is mainly for cleansing purposes, when people are too weak for either the hot or the cold bath.

A Warm Bath is one from 90° to 100° Fahrenheit. This is used especially to relieve sore, stiff joints and muscles after unaccustomed and severe muscular exercise. The bather soaks for some minutes in this bath, which is best taken just before going to bed. Exposure to cold air after such a bath is very likely to result in a cold.

A Hot Bath is one from 100° to 110° Fahrenheit. This is best taken at night also. It is used to prevent a cold after long exposure and to produce sweating. It is good for any one suffering from muscular rheumatism or gout.

A Turkish Bath is a hot-air bath (120° to 170° Fahrenheit), followed by a vigorous shampoo and massage, by various showers and sprays and by a plunge in cold water (60° to 70° Fahrenheit).

A Russian Bath substitutes hot steam (110° to 120° F.), for hot air in the preliminary period.

Turkish and Russian baths are not safe for any one with a weak heart, or who is excessively fat, unless taken on medical advice and under the care of the attendants. In the first stage of a cold they are very valuable, if no subsequent exposure takes place. Rheumatism is often helped by Turkish and Russian baths.

Eating and Drinking.—The proper mode of eating is very important in maintaining good health. Solid food should be thoroughly chewed, not bolted, as the habit is in this age of hurry. It is not well to drink too much fluid with one's meals, as this practice dilutes the digestive juices and may, for that reason, cause indigestion. It is better to drink one or two glasses of water upon rising, again perhaps an hour before luncheon, then late in the afternoon and at night before going to bed. Most people do not drink enough water to keep the secretions in solution and to flush out the organs. A great deal of constipation and some indigestion can be traced to this habit of drinking too little water.

Another modern habit is that of eating too much meat. Once a day is enough to eat meat and twice a day should be the utmost limit. Breakfast is the best time to omit meat. Cereals, bread and fruit are suitable for that meal. At luncheon there may be a small allowance of meat with plenty of vegetables, and then at night a full dinner. In the winter and in a uniformly cold climate people need more meat and fat in their diet than in summer, for meat and fat are great heat-producers. Those who practice severe muscular exertion need an unusual quantity of meat to replace waste of tissue.

There should always be plenty of fruit and fresh vegetables in any diet list. Coffee and tea should be taken in moderation and no healthy person needs alcohol in any form. When raw food is eaten the possibility of taking in parasites, such as various forms of intestinal worms, must be considered. Also the typhoid germ may be taken in from the water in which this raw food has been washed.

Clothing.—A few words must be said on the subject of tight clothing, which restricts the movements of the body. If worn very tight a congestion may be caused, as in the case of wearing tight collars. Severe headache can be traced to this cause. Corsets worn tightly, or even as usually worn, restrict the movement of the ribs and limit the breathing capacity. Unless fitting properly and applied properly, they tend to press the abdominal organs downward.

The amount of clothing should be regulated by the severity of the climate and the exposure the individual undergoes. It is better to be lightly clad in a warm house and then to put on heavy outer wraps when going out. It is a mistake to be too heavily clad indoors, as this causes great sensitiveness to cold, with tendency to sore throats and bronchitis. Garments worn next to the skin should be of some loose-textured substance that absorbs moisture readily and does not give it off too rapidly. Wool is probably the best for this purpose, but cotton underclothing as now manufactured is good enough for all but the very delicate.

It is very dangerous to keep on wet clothes after severe exertion. The rapid cooling of the body due to evaporation may lead to colds, lumbago or even acute kidney disease.

Exercise.—This is very necessary to good health. Every one who leads an active life gets each day a certain amount of exercise. A laborer exercises more than a lawyer, and any one working out of doors will probably get enough exercise and in the best way (that is, without any purpose of exercising). But the majority of people do not get enough muscular exercise, and do not get it in the right way. Exercise should tend to develop the body equally in all parts. No one form does this, hence several methods should be used. A person who walks or runs considerably should row, box or have some gymnasium work which will develop the arms and chest muscles. Rowing, paddling, tennis, baseball and swimming are among the finest of general exercises. But they are too violent for most people. Golf is the best for people as they grow older, for it is milder, and the effort required may be regulated so as to suit the individual, without impairing the skill with which the game is played. Those who can indulge in violent exercise should do so remembering that they are among the fortunate of earth. But most people whose work is not manual labor cannot get such exercise. To them, walking and home gymnastics or developing exercises appeal. There are many excellent systems of easy exercises too numerous to be mentioned in this book.

Home Conditions.—The location of the house is important, especially in the country. High ground is best, with good surface drainage. Low ground, marshy land or clay soil are all unsuitable. A house thus situated is always damp, and rheumatism and bad throat conditions often result. Mosquitoes abound wherever still water is found.

The house itself should be well ventilated, and, as far as possible, all rooms should have sunshine at some time during the day. All living rooms should be thoroughly aired several times during the day.

In moving into a house, it is well to inquire whether consumptives have lived there. The germs of this disease may remain in a house and infect healthy persons. In case of doubt the house should be thoroughly disinfected.

The water supply is very important. In large cities this is carefully looked after by the authorities, but in small places and in the country, each householder must attend to the matter himself. The purity of the supply, and the freedom from contaminating sewage which may cause typhoid, are essential points. The "hard" or "soft" quality of the water is important. Water which is very "hard" contains calcareous salts, which tend to cause constipation, indigestion, and even urinary calculus or "gravel."

HYGIENE OF PREGNANCY

Pregnancy, in itself, is a natural condition and should proceed normally, just as any other function. But, with the advance of civilization, childbearing tends to become more and more pathological, *i. e.* abnormal. Hence, it is the duty of a woman who expects to bear a child, to take such care of herself and to live so correctly during pregnancy as to make the process, if possible, what Nature intended it should be. It is a duty she owes herself and her child. By thought and care during the nine months she is carrying the child, she may save herself great pain and even operative interference at the time of labor.

Clothing.—A pregnant woman should discard all tight clothing as soon as she is aware of her condition. Ordinary corsets should never be worn and her clothes should hang from the shoulders as far as possible. She should wear some thin woolen material next to the skin to avoid taking cold. If the abdomen is large and hangs heavily, some maternity corset or binder should be worn. If the breasts are pendulous and heavy, similar supports should be used.

Low-heeled, common-sense shoes are best and round garters should not be worn. They impede the circulation through the veins.

Exercise.—A moderate amount of daily exercise is the very best thing for a pregnant woman. This should not be indulged in during the period of "morning sickness"; nor should it be carried to the extent of extreme fatigue. But it must be remembered that, in labor, the woman must undergo a severe muscular effort. As in any other form of muscular effort, regular exercise for some time before, best fits the individual to do well. A daily walk in the sunshine, carried just far enough to cause slight fatigue, is the best form during pregnancy. If, for any reason, a patient cannot take this walk, at least let her be in the fresh air for some time each day. All violent exercise, all lifting of heavy weights, and straining of every kind, should be avoided.

Plenty of fresh air day and night should be the rule. The patient is breathing for two, and she needs more oxygen than the normal woman.

Diet.—A woman who is pregnant needs plenty of wholesome and nourishing food, but should avoid all rich, indigestible articles of diet. She should drink plenty of water, milk or cocoa. Tea and coffee should be taken in moderation and alcoholic drinks *not at all*. Sometimes the woman craves unusual food. Such craving should be respected in most cases, because it reveals the need of the body for the particular elements which that food contains.

As pregnancy advances, the amount of food eaten at one time becomes less. This is due to the enlarging uterus, which presses upward on the stomach. Hence light meals should be given between the larger meals. The mother must eat to maintain her own strength and her child's.

If there is any suggestion of kidney trouble or severe vomiting, the diet must be altered considerably. But the doctor in charge will attend to that.

Bowels.—Constipation is to be avoided. To eliminate properly all waste products is most important for a normal pregnancy. Plenty of water should be taken, the coarser cereals and vegetables should be chosen, and if necessary a daily dose of some laxative given. Compound Licorice Powder or Cascara is best. Salts are not recommended except for very occasional use.

Massage.—If a woman will begin to massage her breasts and nipples daily after the sixth or seventh month, she will find, when she comes to nurse her baby, that her skin will be in much better condition. Cocoa-butter, olive oil or vaseline may be used to advantage for this purpose. Many women have suffered severely from cracked and tender nipples. Care and a little trouble on their part would have saved them much pain.

Mental Condition.—Pregnancy affects the mental condition of women differently. Some continue very much as before, but others suffer from mental depression, are suspicious and unhappy, and, in fact, almost seem to change their natures. Such patients should be protected from all worries and annoyances, their spells of irritation overlooked, and everything done to make them happy.

It is a duty which every woman owes herself and her unborn child to place herself in a doctor's care as soon as she becomes aware of her pregnancy.

As the time draws near for the labor, a woman should have everything for herself and the baby in readiness. The nurse and the doctor should be engaged and the room prepared. Then, the last days before labor may be spent in peace, the best preparation for the severe strain ahead.

HYGIENE OF PUBERTY

Puberty is that period in a child's life when the boy begins to be a man and the girl begins to be a woman. In the boy the change is marked by the deepened voice, the growth of hair on the face and a coarsening and enlarging of the features. In the girl, there comes a softening and rounding of contour, the body develops, the girl feels an increased modesty and shyness, and, most important of all, the function of menstruation is established.

Menstruation is the monthly discharge of blood and secretions from the uterus. It begins usually between the ages of twelve and fifteen. Some children begin even earlier and a few later. The discharge occurs every twenty-eight or thirty days and lasts from two to five days. This is a delicate period, when the whole system is undergoing a change; the girl's nerves and mind are very sensitive and easily unstrung. No strain, physical or mental, should be put on a girl for a year or so, for this is the danger period. At such a time, bad habits are easily formed, and the results of strain are marked on the impressionable brain and the plastic body.

This is the period when a girl should be kept from severe exercise. Her sexual organs are developing and are very susceptible to injury. Heavy lifting, straining or jumping often result in a displacement of these organs, which may cause the girl suffering for years. Nature did not intend that women should suffer pain and be unable to work at their monthly periods. Civilization and luxurious living have brought about this condition. But, to a large extent, a mother, by training her daughter in correct habits, may bring the child back to the normal standard.

Whenever possible, a girl should rest quietly the first day of her sickness. Her clothing should be loose and warm; corsets should not be worn. There is usually a tendency to constipation at the menstrual period. This should be overcome by a good dose of some saline cathartic, the day before the period is expected. Do not take any pills containing aloin, for that drug aggravates the uterine cramps.

At first, it is best not to take any baths during the period. But as a girl gets older and the function is established normally, there is no objection to a daily sponge in warm water, provided there is no exposure to cold.

No violent exercise should be allowed during the entire period in a young girl.

Between periods a girl should take plenty of moderate exercise in the open air. Tennis and such extremely violent athletics are best given up for a few years. Clothing should be sensible and loose. The child should have plenty of good plain food, but all rich, indigestible food should be avoided and there should be no eating between meals. Nothing so quickly upsets a child's general condition as promiscuous eating at all hours of the day.

At this developing period, no girl should be forced in her studies. It would be better to take her out of school entirely, than to crowd her with work. It is a small matter if a girl drops back a class at such a time. She will more than counterbalance the loss by the avoidance of ill health.

Every mother is confronted with the question: How much shall I tell my daughter about the subject of sex and child-bearing? Each one must decide the question for herself, but a word of advice is not out of place. Every girl who has arrived at the time of puberty has a right to know certain simple facts, for her own protection. If her mother does not tell her these, properly and correctly, her schoolmates will tell them improperly and incorrectly. Many a girl has felt like reproaching her mother when she has looked back at childhood and realized how different her situation might have been if she had received proper instruction from her mother. Many good books have been written for girls on this subject, and any woman may safely put such a book in her daughter's hands and let her learn for herself the essential facts of life.

CHAPTER III

FIRST AID

The subject of First Aid to the Injured is especially important. In sudden accidents immediate treatment is most needed, and usually in these cases it is most difficult to get a doctor promptly. An attempt has been made to cover the whole field of probable accidents and to outline briefly their dangers and the proper treatment. Although we do not continually reiterate the advice to seek a physician as soon as possible, it must be understood that after "first aid" has been rendered, we assume that medical advice will be sought. We shall take up the different accidents under separate headings.

REVIVING THE DROWNED

When There Is More Than One Assistant

General Rules

Rule 1. Arouse the patient if possible, by exposing his face to the air at once, loosening his clothing, and quickly slapping his chest with the flat of the hand. If his condition does not change, then do as follows:

Rule 2. Expel the water from the stomach and chest. First get the jaws open and insert some sort of a mouth gag, such as a small piece of wood, a cork, or a pencil with a handkerchief wrapped about it. Turn the patient face downwards and place some object under the stomach. A large bundle of clothes, a box, a log—any object near at hand will do. Then proceed to press heavily on the back of the patient for about a minute, or as long as fluids flow freely from the mouth.

Rule 3: Artificial Respiration to Produce Breathing: Turn patient on back and elevate that portion of the body between the hips and the shoulders. Get the chin forward and the head as far back as possible. Clear the throat of mucus by wrapping any sort of cloth about the forefinger and swabbing it out. Then grasp the tongue between the thumb and forefinger (it is easier to hold the tongue with a handkerchief or piece of cloth) and pull it out of one corner of the mouth. This prevents choking and makes it possible for the patient to breathe.

Another assistant should grasp the arms, just below the elbows, and draw them steadily upward by the sides of the patient's head to the ground,

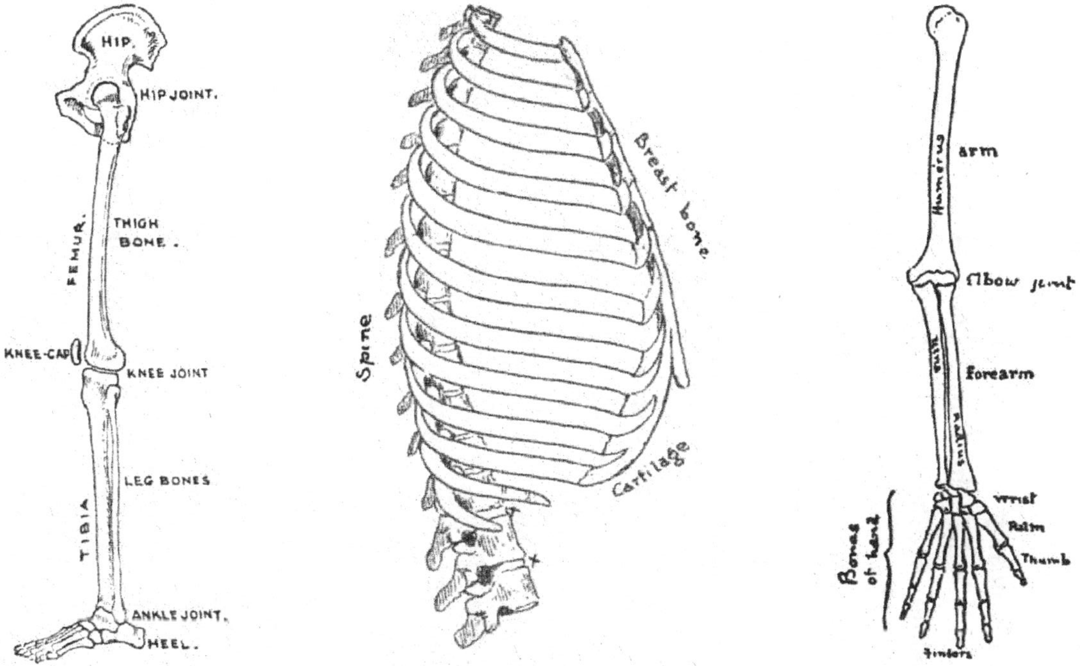

BONES OF THE LEG, CHEST AND ARM

the hands nearly meeting. This act enlarges the capacity of the chest and induces inspiration. Meanwhile, another assistant gets astride of the patient and stands ready with his hands on him; the balls of the thumbs resting on either side of that part of the body below the ribs, the fingers falling into the grooves between the short ribs. When the hands of the patient are taken from above his head and brought down at his sides to the ground, the last assistant will put all his weight forward on his hands and at the same time squeeze the waist between them. He will keep pressing deeper and deeper for about five seconds, when, with a final push, he will cease and the assistant with the arms will again proceed to draw them above the head.

These movements should be repeated from twelve to fifteen times a minute. If, after trying this for about five minutes, breathing does not occur, turn the patient on his stomach and try to expel more water. Then practice artificial respiration again. Do not give up, for you may save the patient after doing artificial respiration for three hours. If possible, have the body rubbed while trying to revive the patient. Rub vigorously and always in the direction of the heart. Get heat to the extremities if possible. If a physician is near at hand, call him at once. By so doing you may save a life.

RULE 4. Treatment After Patient Breathes: After the breathing is established, see that the patient is dry and put him in a dry, warm place with fresh air to breathe. If he is very weak, a stimulant, such as a half ounce or an ounce of whisky or brandy, may be given; but the better plan is to get a physician, who will give heart and respiratory stimulants. A physician is especially required, since congestion of the lungs is very liable to follow such an exposure.

When There is Only One Person to Revive the Patient.—A new method called "The Pressure Prone Method" has lately been devised by the English Coast Guards, and has been enthusiastically adopted by practically all life-saving stations. It is very simple and its greatest value lies in the fact that only one person is needed to do it. A description follows:

Place the patient on his stomach with his head on one side, so that air can reach his nose and mouth. Let the head and upper part of the body be a little lower than the legs if possible. Gravity will then cause the water to run out of the lungs and also gravity will keep the jaw forward and the tongue in place.

Next kneel astride the patient (as in the diagram), facing the head. Of course, if the patient is a woman, loosen all tight clothing and cut the corsets. Then place your hands, palm down and thumbs toward the centre, over the lower ribs near the middle of the back. Next throw your whole body weight on your hands, pressing down and squeezing it while you count one, two, slowly—almost a second for each. Then suddenly slacken pressure and lift your hands while you count three. Then repeat the whole process. When you press down, you expel some water and air from the lungs by diminishing the space in them. When your weight is removed, atmospheric pressure drives the air in to fill up the increased space caused by the elastic expansion of the lungs. Any one can readily see that this method can be kept up for hours by one person. The position is easy and no great strength is required. Even if other people are present, it is the better method, and the other people may be kept busy applying heat to the extremities, rubbing arms and legs, etc. After breathing has been re-established, the treatment is the same as given above.

HEAT PROSTRATION AND SUNSTROKE

The symptoms of these two conditions and the

treatment of each are entirely different. It is important to be able to differentiate between Heat Prostration or Exhaustion, and Sunstroke.

Heat Prostration.—This is caused by overwork, worry or poor food, combined with exposure to severe heat, and great physical exertion. One does not have to be exposed to the direct rays of the sun to suffer. In out-of-door workers the attack usually begins in the afternoon or early evening.

SYMPTOMS.—Sense of weakness, dizziness, restlessness, headache. Then the skin becomes pale, cool and moist. This condition is very often preceded by profuse sweating. The prostration is great, pulse rapid and weak, breathing feeble with lowered temperature, often 97° or 95° Fahrenheit. As a rule, the person remains conscious.

TREATMENT.—1. Get the patient in a cool place (shady, if out-of-doors) and lay him flat on his back. Loosen all tight clothing. If in the city call an ambulance or a private physician. If neither can be had, give patient half a cup of clear, strong, black coffee.

2. Put the patient to bed and keep him there until the doctor sees him. In a few hours recovery will be complete.

Sunstroke.—This is a very serious condition.

Workers in the open under a hot sun are susceptible. The habitual use of alcohol makes the individual more liable to this condition. The attack is often preceded by a cessation of sweating. This should always warn a man of coming trouble.

SYMPTOMS.—The attack is ushered in with dizziness, violent pains in the head, spots appearing before the eyes, nausea and retching. The patient soon becomes comatose. The face is red, the breathing is loud and hard, pulse is bounding, the muscles, as a rule, are relaxed, but there may be twitching followed by convulsions. The temperature runs high, 105° to 107° Fahrenheit by mouth; by rectum it may go up to 112° Fahrenheit. After observing the "first-aid" laws, get a physician.

TREATMENT.—1. Call an ambulance or a physician if in a city. Be sure to get medical advice, if possible.

2. Remove to a shady spot. Loosen all tight clothing. Strip naked and place on canvas if possible.

3. Sprinkle or bathe with ice-water or apply cold cloths.

4. If a sheet is handy, soak it in ice-water and wrap it about a patient, keeping it wet with ice-water. Place a bit of ice, wrapped in a cloth, back of the neck.

5. When the temperature falls nearly to normal, put to bed with an ice-cap on the head. The physician will give stimulation and enemas.

WOUNDS

A wound or laceration is a cut or tear of the skin alone or of the skin and deeper structures of the body.

In all lacerations of the body, if the flow of blood is easily checked and the deeper structures are not involved, the treatment is very simple, yet of vital importance. If dirt is in the wound, clean it out with water that has been boiled, or hot water with ordinary table salt added to it. A teaspoonful of salt to a pint of water is the proportion to use. After cleansing the laceration to the best of your ability, apply a wet dressing and bandage. An antiseptic tablet should be dissolved in warm water, and the dressings soaked in it. Keep the bandage wet from one to two days. Then use dry dressings. The important thing is to have all dressings clean and germ-proof. If the laceration is a long or deep one, or if it occurs on the scalp and the patient is dazed, or bleeds from the mouth, nose or ears, call a physician, as the patient will require expert attention, to determine whether his skull is fractured. Accompanying a slight cut on a head, very often there is a fractured skull.

If, after two or three days, the structures around the part involved are swollen, red, or give off heat, or if pus is in evidence, do not attempt to treat it yourself. Use wet antiseptic dressings and call a physician. He may save a hand, arm or leg, or possibly a life. The average individual does not seem to realize the dangers of an infected wound.

Bleeding from an Artery.—This is easily recognized. The blood spurts from the wound and is of a bright red color. Sometimes a cut artery will spurt blood five feet. The first-aid laws are: Do things quickly. Make firm pressure with the fingers between the wound and the heart. Pressure directly over the bleeding point will stop the flow of blood. If the artery cut is in an extremity, pass around the extremity, between the wound and the heart, any cord-like object, such as a rope, strap, string, rubber tubing or suspenders, and tie the ends; then put a stick, rod, cane or umbrella through the noose you have made and twist up the slack until the bleeding stops. Do not keep this pressure on for more than half an hour at a time. Gangrene may result. Send for medical aid immediately, as it is essential for a surgeon to pick up and tie the bleeding vessel.

Bleeding from a Vein.—This is readily recognized by the steady flow of dark blood. It is easy to stop and it is not necessary to tie the vessel. Apply pressure directly over the bleeding vein itself, or between the wound and the extremity; that is, on the side of the cut away from the heart. Bandage snugly and remove dressings in about a half hour and see if bleeding has stopped. If so, re-apply bandage, but more loosely. Too much pressure, continued for more than an hour or two, will cause pain and may do serious damage. Keep the wounded part warm with hot water bottles or coverings. If the flow of blood is very profuse or persistent call a physician.

Bleeding from Punctured Wounds.—First remove any foreign body, such as a pin, tack or splinter; then clean and apply a wet antiseptic dressing. If the wound becomes red and painful, call a physician, as it probably will need to be opened in order that good drainage may be established. If caused by a bullet, rusty nail or gunpowder, seek medical aid at once, as lockjaw is liable to follow.

General Oozing of Blood from a Raw Surface.—Unless a person is a "bleeder," general oozing is readily checked by applying water as hot as the person can stand, elevating the part injured and

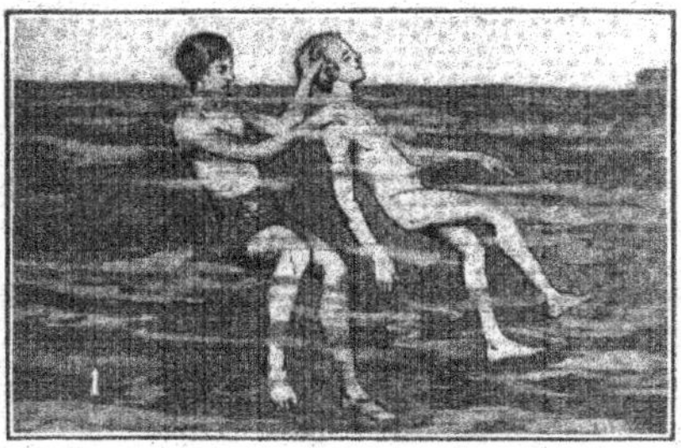

Seize him by hair and shoulders

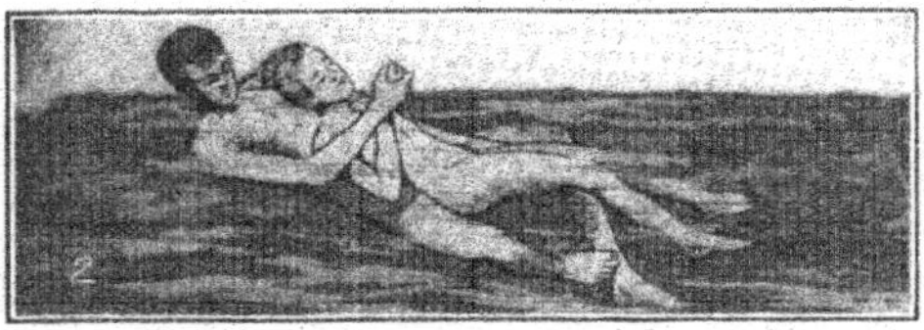

Grasp his hand

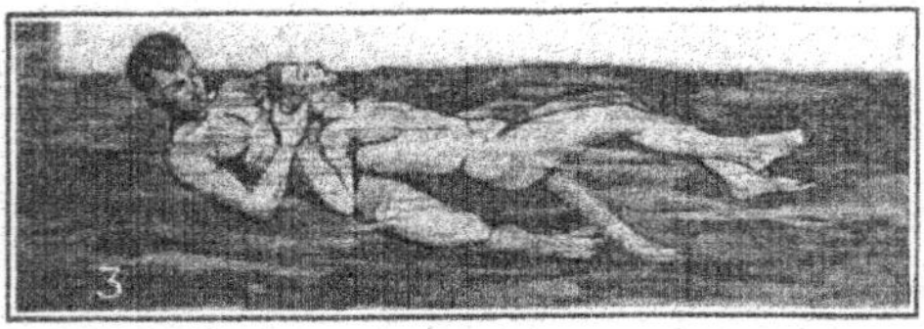

And draw him onto your chest

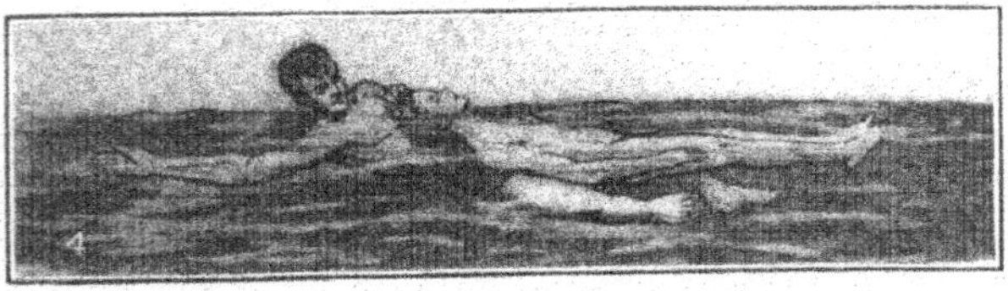

Holding him by the hair, swim on your back

BRINGING A DROWNING PERSON TO SHORE

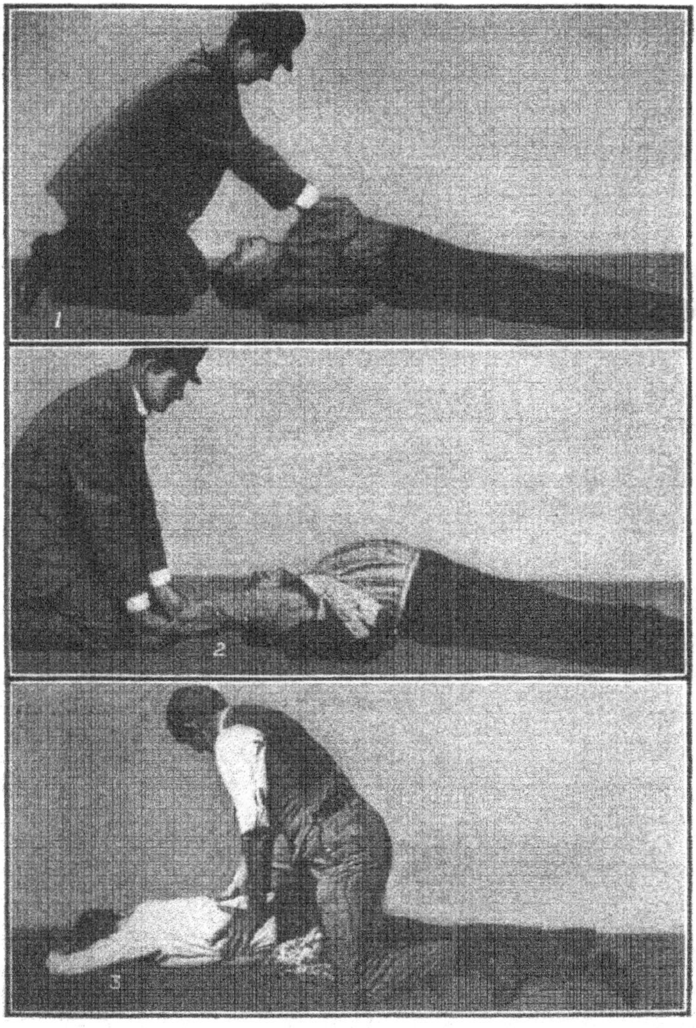

1 AND 2. THE SYLVESTER METHOD OF ARTIFICIAL RESPIRATION
3. THE PRESSURE PRONE METHOD OF ARTIFICIAL RESPIRATION
(See article on Reviving the Drowned)

applying a tight wet bandage. If a person is a "bleeder" and the oozing cannot be stopped, call a doctor.

Bleeding from Scalp.—A scalp wound bleeds profusely. Therefore, do not be alarmed at the sight of a head covered with blood.

When a person has a scalp wound and a physician is not near at hand, cut the hair off surrounding the wound and apply a dressing of some antiseptic solution (See Appendix), or if procurable, swab the wound with Pure Tincture of Iodine. Put a clean piece of linen or gauze directly over the wound and bandage.

Nose-Bleed.—In nose-bleeds have the patient sit erect and apply ice to the nape of the neck. Press finger firmly against the upper lip. Apply pressure to lower edge of jaw bone about one inch in front of the angle of the jaw, thus compressing the facial artery, which supplies the nose. Do not remove the clots. If the bleeding continues, soak a strip of gauze in vinegar and plug the nose. This will often arrest bleeding. If the bleeding is profuse and cannot be stopped, call a physician, who will plug the posterior nares or back of throat.

For bleeding from lungs and stomach, see chapter treating diseases of the respiratory and digestive systems.

Electric Shock or Lightning Stroke.—If the patient is still in contact with the live wire, great care must be exercised to protect oneself. If it is possible to shut off the current, do so. But if not, protect your hands with heavy, *dry* leather or rubber gloves, or else pry the patient off with a *dry* stick. Anything wet conducts electricity very easily.

Symptoms.—General muscular contractions, faintness and unconsciousness, failure of pulse and breathing. Continued unconsciousness is a favorable symptom. Very often there is a loss of muscular power. Burns of all degrees occur at the points of entrance and exit of the current.

Treatment.—First break the contact or have the current shut off. If the heart has stopped, the case is fatal and nothing can be done. If the patient is not dead, artificial respiration (see directions for Reviving the Drowned) is the most valuable remedy and should be continued for hours. A physician should be called to give the proper stimulation. While waiting for a physician, a rectal injection of whisky—two tablespoonfuls in a cup of warm water—or strong black coffee is advantageous. A mustard plaster (see Appendix), placed over the heart may be tried with good results. Keep the body warm with blankets and place hot water bottles against the extremities. The burns should be cleansed and dressed surgically.

Shock and Collapse.—Shock is a sudden depression of the vital centres arising from an injury or a profound emotion, acting on the nerve centres and inducing exhaustion. (From Da Costa's *Modern Surgery.*)

The blood in the arteries and capillaries goes to the veins. Therefore, there is a deficient amount of blood in circulation.

The term "collapse" is used by some to designate a severe condition of shock and is employed by others as a name for a condition of shock produced by mental disturbance rather than physical injury.

Shock may be slight and pass by quickly, or it may be severe and prolonged, even producing death.

Shock is more severe in women than in men.

Causes.—Fear, injuries of the nerves, of the brain, of the organs of the chest and abdomen, kidney diseases, diabetes, heart disease, anything which extracts the body-heat, such as exposure to cold air, cerebral concussion, or sudden and profuse hemorrhage. Shock also occurs after certain surgical operations and the exposure of tissue and vital parts to the air. Certain poisons have this effect, also.

SYMPTOMS.—The temperature is sub-normal, and the pulse is irregular, weak and rapid; the skin is cold, pallid and clammy, with profuse perspiration and irregular, shallow breathing. Consciousness is usually retained, but there is an absence of mental originating power. The pupils are dilated and react slowly to light. Pain is either slight or not felt at all. Nausea is absent, but there may be vomiting. Gastric regurgitation is a bad sign, and if delirium occurs the condition is grave. There is often a suppression of urine and the bowels move involuntarily.

TREATMENT.—1. Place the patient flat on his back.

2. Raise feet and lower the head, unless blueness of face occurs.

3. Wrap patient in blankets and apply hot water bottles or bricks. (See chapter on Home Nursing.)

4. Ordinary stimulants are of little value and drugs given by stomach are not absorbed. Salt solution per rectum or enemas of hot coffee and whisky are valuable. (See chapter on Home Nursing.)

5. Bandage the extremities.

6. Apply a compress or a binder tightly to the abdomen. It helps to drive out the imprisoned blood.

7. Put mustard plasters over heart, spine and shins.

Fainting.—Many different conditions cause fainting. The first-aid treatment is the same, regardless of the cause:

1. Loosen all clothing.

2. Put a pad or cushion under the hips and raise the feet. This does not apply if the face is flushed or congested. But most patients are pale when in a faint.

3. Put ammonia water or smelling salts under the nose.

4. Spatter cold water on face.

5. Give one teaspoonful of aromatic spirits of ammonia in water.

6. As soon as the patient can be moved, get him to bed with hot water bags about him and keep him quiet.

Suffocation from Gas in Wells, Cisterns or Mines, or from Illuminating Gas.—

TREATMENT.—1. Get to pure air.

2. Resuscitate as if drowned. (See Directions for Reviving the Drowned.) Keep the body warm.

3. Give saline enemas. (See chapter on Home Nursing.)

4. Seek medical aid.

Fit or Convulsion.—

TREATMENT.—1. Loosen all clothing, especially corsets.

2. Restrain; thereby protecting patient from injury.

3. Protect the tongue from being bitten. Use a mouth gag, such as a cork, or rubber eraser, tied to a string.

4. Let patient sleep after fit without rousing.

Concussion of Brain.—This condition occurs as a result of a severe fall or blow on the head. The brain tissue is severely shaken up without being lacerated or wounded.

SYMPTOMS.—The patient is usually dazed, stupid and unable to locate himself or realize what has happened. When he recovers, in the course of a few hours, he has no recollection of his accident or subsequent conduct.

TREATMENT.—Protect the patient from injury if he is violent and keep him quiet until he recovers spontaneously. There is little to do except to put an ice bag on the head, and to keep the patient quiet. A teaspoonful of aromatic spirits of ammonia may be given in a little water.

Contusions.—A contusion is a bruise. Some contusions amount to nothing, others are severe enough to need treatment.

Symptoms.—Immediately following the blow, the part struck becomes swollen and darkened. This is because blood vessels have been ruptured and blood is leaking out into the tissues. This leaking may be considerable, so that a large clot of blood is collected. Unless the skin is cut by a doctor and this clot expressed out, it must be absorbed. Often the clot becomes infected by some germ and an abscess results. The skin over the contusion is also bruised and blood oozes through it. It becomes discolored by the blood pigment and we have the typical "black and blue" marks. When the muscle is involved in the contusion, it becomes very sore and all motion or use of that muscle causes pain. Sometimes weeks are required to absorb completely the blood which has oozed out.

Treatment.—Immediately following the blow, bathe the part in cold water and apply an ice bag. This will keep the swelling down. After an hour or so of such treatment, begin applying hot water to the part to prevent discoloration as far as possible. Massage gently for a few minutes every night and morning. This will hasten absorption.

Burns and Scalds.—A burn is caused by dry heat and a scald by moist heat.

Burns are usually classed as of three degrees. In a first-degree burn, the skin is reddened, but not blistered or broken, and only the outer layer of skin is injured. In a second-degree burn there are blisters and the whole skin is involved in the burn. A third-degree burn is where charring or complete destruction has taken place.

In addition to the pain, a burn causes severe shock.

TREATMENT.—When there is no blister or broken skin, cover all the burned area with thick cloths wet in a strong solution of baking soda. Keep these dressings wet continually and do not let the burned area come in contact with the air. If the pain is intense and no doctor can be reached, it is safe to give a teaspoonful of paregoric. Do not repeat the dose until the doctor has arrived. For a child, divide this dose in half.

If there are blisters, do not break them; the doctor will do that, using proper antiseptic precautions. If the blisters have already ruptured do not let the raw surface be exposed to dirt. Cover with clean cloths as soon as possible. The first-aid treatment for this class is the same as for the first class. A saturated solution of baking soda is used to wet the cloths which are laid over the burns. This is cooling and keeps out the air. Keep these dressings wet continually. To counteract the shock give black coffee (see Home Nursing), or aromatic spirits of ammonia, a teaspoonful to a glass of water; apply hot-water bags to the feet, and give paregoric (a teaspoonful) for the pain. The burned person is usually very thirsty. He should have ice to hold in his mouth, cold milk and water to drink.

If the burns are extensive or the shock is great, the patient should be put to bed. If wet dressings are used, it is best to put him directly on a rubber or oilcloth sheet. Do not put any night-shirt or pajamas on him, as these only cause pain on their removal, or when the daily dressings are renewed. Cover the patient warmly, but have the covers raised, so that their weight does not give unnecessary pain. Keep the bowels well opened with soap-suds enemas, and, especially in a man, note carefully whether he passes his urine after the injury. If he does not do this within twelve hours, medical aid must be obtained, for the patient will have to be catheterized; if this is not done, rupture of the bladder may occur.

In third-degree burns, the shock is usually the most important feature and should be treated first.

The patient must be stimulated with doses of whisky, an ounce to half a glass of water, by mouth, or an ounce in a hot-coffee enema. Apply heat to the extremities. The first dressings are the same as described in first-degree burns. Later, the destroyed flesh will soften and slough off. Its removal may be hastened by cutting the loose ends away with scissors.

Other Methods of Treatment.—A good emergency material to be used is the thick lather of any ordinary hand-soap. This is to be obtained almost anywhere. Make a thick lather, smear it over the burns, and then apply dressings and bandages.

Carron oil (equal parts of linseed oil and lime water) is an old and well known dressing for burns. There are many objections to its use. It is not sterile, and may contain many germs which will infect the raw surface of a burn, besides being very dirty. But, for burns with an unbroken skin, its use is permissible.

Burns by Strong Acid.—Neutralize the acid by applying an alkali dissolved in water. Baking soda or lime-water is efficacious and can usually be obtained. Very weak ammonia (about a teaspoonful to a pint) will also serve. Then wash off thoroughly with water and dress like any other burn.

Burns by Strong Alkali (*Potash or Strong Ammonia*).—Neutralize by pouring vinegar or a very weak acid over the surface. Then wash and dress the burn. Do not use baking soda for this, as it is alkaline. Use a solution of boric acid.

Frost-Bite and Freezing.—The nose, fingers, ears and toes are usually affected. But in severe cases, the whole body is more or less involved and the patient may be unconscious. The parts frozen are numb, stiff, pale or blue.

TREATMENT.—The object is to restore the body heat and circulation. This must be done slowly or the results may be fatal. Keep the person in a cold room and rub the frosted parts gently with snow or cold water. Gradually the rubbing may become more vigorous. As the circulation returns rub with alcohol and water and gradually increase the heat of the room.

If the patient stops breathing, use artificial respiration. (See Reviving the Drowned.) While one person does this (for several hours, if necessary), others must keep up the rubbing and massage. If any part of the skin becomes permanently dead through freezing, it will slough off. This is treated exactly as if it were a burn.

When the circulation is restored and breathing is re-established, warm stimulating drinks, such as hot black coffee, should be given, the patient put to bed and kept warm and quiet.

Frost-bite is a superficial freezing and is of varying severity. The treatment is the same as for freezing. Rub with snow or cold water in a cold room. The parts frozen usually recover completely with only a slight peeling. In other cases, the skin completely sloughs away.

Chilblains.—This is an inflammation which often follows freezing or frost-bite. It will sometimes recur for years at every return of cold weather. The parts swell, become red, are attended by burning, itching and smarting.

TREATMENT.—People susceptible to chilblains should always wear thick woolen stockings and gloves. When chilled, one should not enter a warm room too suddenly, but should warm up slowly. Daily cold baths help this condition. For the itching, treat as described in Skin Diseases.

How to Diagnose Death.—Legally death is not certain until signs of decomposition set in. But, practically there are several ways of being sure the patient has expired. The old method of holding the watch crystal to the mouth and nose and noting whether it clouds over with the moisture of the breath, is very inaccurate. Of course, as long as breathing or the beating of the heart can be detected, we know the patient is alive. But, even when we cannot detect these signs of vitality, the spark of life may still be present. The best method is to feel the eyeball. During life this has a certain tension easily determined by feeling one's own eye with the lid closed. In a few minutes after death the eyeball softens, and on pressure does not present the firm feeling characteristic of a living eye. It remains indented at the point of pressure. If this result is obtained by experiment, death is practically certain.

Dislocations.—A dislocation is, popularly, the putting out of joint of some part of the body, as the elbow or shoulder. Anatomically, one of the articulating bones of a joint has been forced out of its normal position.

When the displacement is momentary, and the bone returns immediately to its place, the accident is called a *sprain.*

There are three principal classes of dislocations:

1. Traumatic dislocations; the result of direct or indirect violence, from muscular action.

2. Pathological dislocations; due to slow changes in the ligaments and tissues of the joint, muscular action being the active agent in causing the ultimate displacement.

3. Congenital dislocations which result from

imperfect development of the joint in infancy and childhood.

We are concerned here only with the first class or traumatic dislocations. Three dislocations out of every four involve some joint of the arm or hand, and among these, dislocation of the shoulder is most frequent.

If the skin which covers a dislocated joint is penetrated, the dislocation is known as a "compound dislocation." This condition is rare and should be treated as a wound; absolute rest of the injured member should be assured and medical aid swiftly sought.

Symptoms of Dislocations.—1. The deformity of the joint discloses the nature of the injury in many cases.

2. The normal range of motion of the limb is restricted.

3. Pain is present in all cases, especially when the limb is moved or the injured part handled. The persistence of severe pain indicates that some of the soft parts near the joint are not torn, but are kept forcibly stretched.

4. The normal outline or contour of the region about the affected joint is changed.

5. The direction of the axis of the dislocated bone is altered.

The swelling that takes place about the larger joints makes it difficult to distinguish a fracture from a dislocation. This is for the surgeon, who must be summoned at once.

Many people seem to have but one idea when a person has a dislocation; that is, to grasp the limb and pull. Harm often results from this procedure. In order to reduce the dislocation successfully the anatomy of the injured part must be known.

Therefore, it is wise to postpone the attempt to reduce the dislocation until the doctor arrives.

There are three common dislocations that sometimes can be reduced without medical aid. Even with these, it is better to call a physician, but if none is at hand, the following instructions may be useful.

Dislocation of Lower Jaw.—One side or frequently both sides are affected, with the displacement forward.

It is frequent in women and rare in children and in the aged.

SYMPTOMS.—The jaw is rigid and it is impossible to close the mouth. The chin projects forward. A deviation of the jaw toward the uninjured side is observed in one-sided dislocations.

TREATMENT.—Depress the angle of the jaw, and

support the chin at the same time. Pull the jaw bone down until it slips into its socket. After this, the joint should be kept as quiet as possible for two weeks at least.

Shoulder Joint.—The displacements may be either upward, outward, downward, inward, backward, or forward.

In the inward variety, the vessels and nerves are more likely to be disturbed by pressure.

Symptoms.—Pain is present in the affected region. The shoulder is flattened and there is a depression of the skin over the cavity. There is a lengthening of the arm in the forward, downward and backward displacements and shortening of the arm in the upward displacement.

The elbow cannot be carried inward or forward on the chest, and the hand cannot be placed on the opposite shoulder while the elbow is lifted.

Treatment.—Only when it is impossible to get medical aid for days, should an attempt be made to correct the dislocation.

The anterior or forward dislocation is the most common variety and the most efficient method of reduction is known as the Kocher's rotation method, which is used in the following manner:

The elbow is carried to the side, with the forearm at right angles to the arm; and the arm is then forcibly rotated until the forearm points away from the body. When this is done, the arm is carried up from the body until it is in the horizontal position. When the arm comes to the level of the shoulder, it is gradually rotated, and is again brought to the side with the forearm across the body. The head of the bone slips into place with the inward rotation, and at the beginning of the downward movement. The method requires great care, especially when applied to the aged. After the dislocation has been reduced, bandage or strap the arm to the chest.

Thumb Dislocation.—The dislocation backward is less frequent than forward. Sometimes it is easily reduced, but often great difficulty is experienced in correcting the deformity, and not infrequently a surgical operation has to be performed.

TREATMENT.—Press the thumb backward and at the same time attempt to lift the head of the bone into its socket.

Fractures.—A fracture is the breaking of a bone or cartilage.

SYMPTOMS.—The signs of a fracture are easily recognized when the break is complete. A cracked bone, or a bone broken part way, is not so easily detected.

TREATMENT.—Never attempt to set a fracture.

Keep the fragments of bone from being moved, by applying a splint, and try to make the patient comfortable. A surgeon should be called to treat the fracture. There are, however, several first-aid laws to be observed.

In compound fractures (that is, where the skin is ruptured by the broken bone), if the bleeding is severe and does not stop, treat as in any bleeding. (See article on Bleeding.)

If the bleeding has stopped, or is not severe, keep the injured part absolutely quiet and wash the wound with hot water. Then, shave a large area about the wound and apply clean dressings.

If a rib is fractured, have the patient put his hands on his head, and let out his breath; then apply a piece of adhesive plaster, about a foot wide and two feet long, tightly over the injured part and around the body.

In the case of a fractured collar-bone put the patient flat on his back with the arm at the side, the elbow bent and the hand resting on the opposite side of the chest. Then, put a heavy weight (*e. g.* a sand bag) on the broken bone.

In a fracture of the lower jaw, press the fragments into place and bandage the lower jaw firmly against the upper jaw.

In a fracture of the arm, wrap two pieces of

wood, or stiff cardboard, eight by three inches, separately, with cloths or handkerchiefs. Carefully bring the broken parts together, apply the padded splints on each side of the fracture and bandage tightly. Then, put the arm in a sling.

It is better to wait several hours for trained medical aid, than for an unskilful person to attempt to correct the injury.

In fracture of a finger, apply splints and bandage.

In fracture of a hip, put the patient flat on his back, with the injured limb between pillows, until a surgeon arrives.

In fracture of the thigh-bone, get a board which will reach from the ankle to the armpit, pad it if possible and bandage it fast to the leg and body. The hollow between the splint and the waist must be filled with padding before the bandage is applied.

In kneepan fracture, place a splint the length of the limb behind the leg and the bed. Fill the space behind the knee with padding and apply bandages above and below the knee. Keep cold wet sponges or cracked ice on the knee.

In fracture of the bones of the leg, between the knee and the ankle, be very careful in handling.

Prepare two splints, one large and heavy, long

enough to extend from the ankle to three or five inches above the knee. Apply the lighter splint on the outer side of the leg and place the heavy splint on the back of the leg. Fasten the splints with bandages.

When the ankle joint is fractured, attempt to correct the deformity, if such appears. Then apply splints, extending from the soles of the feet to the knee on either side of the ankle, and bandage.

Sprains.—A sprain is caused by a sudden wrench or twist, experienced most frequently in the ankle and wrist.

SYMPTOMS.—The symptoms are severe pain, swelling, arrested movement, tenderness and heat of the injured parts. After the first attack, there occurs a period of comparative ease, followed, either quickly or more commonly after a lapse of some hours, by a return of the suffering, due to the tension and inflammation.

TREATMENT.—In mild cases, rest, with cold or hot applications, may be all that is required.

Compression is of great value. Wrap a layer of cotton or wool around the joint and hold it in place by a moderately tight bandage of flannel. After the active inflammation has subsided, massage is of great value. Unless the sprain is a trifle, consult a surgeon.

Surgical Dressings.—Any clean, "antiseptic" cotton, lint or gauze may be used for dressings. Freshly washed and ironed goods may be used in an emergency.

Bandaging is an art in itself, and a book might be written giving a description of the various methods of applying a bandage.

Use common sense, and let the bandage cover the injured part. Any bandage which stays on is successful.

Ingrowing Toe-nails.—Ingrowing toe-nails are caused by the wearing of improper shoes, causing pressure, or a wrong method of cutting the nails, which gives rise to a condition in which the flesh along the edges of the toe-nail becomes inflamed.

Toe-nails should be cut straight across, and not trimmed too closely at the corners.

SYMPTOMS.—The flesh about the nail becomes red, tender, painful and swollen, so that it overlaps the nail. Pus may form. Wearing a shoe or walking becomes difficult. The condition may last for months, if not properly treated.

TREATMENT.—Wear broad-toed shoes, with low heels.

Hot poultices will relieve the pain and inflammation.

Soak the foot in hot water and push the flesh

back from the nail. An antiseptic powder should be dusted along the edge of the nail.

If pus forms or the condition persists, consult a surgeon.

Emergency Treatment in Childbirth.—It sometimes happens that a doctor does not arrive until after a baby is born or else no doctor can be obtained immediately. For the safety of both mother and child, certain things must be done.

When the baby is delivered, it must be made to breathe, if it does not do so spontaneously. Hold it up by the feet, with a towel to prevent slipping, and slap its back rather vigorously. Wipe the baby's mouth to get rid of the mucus which may have collected. Spank the buttocks smartly and then splash hot and cold water alternately on the chest and back. If breathing does not begin, lay the baby down and perform artificial respiration.

The umbilical cord connects the child with the placenta or "afterbirth." This must be tied and cut, but do not hurry about this until the child's breathing is established. Take any clean, strong cord or narrow tape, and boil it if there is time. Tie the cord in two places about two inches apart and about two inches from the baby. Then cut between the ties. Watch the end connected with the baby for bleeding. If there is any bleeding, re-tie more tightly. Then, pour a little alcohol over the stump, put a piece of clean gauze or cotton on it and a snug binder passing round the baby's body.

As soon as the baby has been delivered, some one should rub the mother's abdomen vigorously. A hard, firm mass will be felt under the skin. This is the womb or uterus, which still contains the afterbirth. This should be rubbed vigorously until the afterbirth is expelled. Then it should be held firmly. As long as this is hard and firm there is little danger of hemorrhage. But, if it softens up, there will be bleeding. As soon as softness is felt, rub with increased vigor until the womb hardens again. Send to the nearest drug store and get some fluid extract of ergot, explaining for what it is to be used. Give the mother a teaspoonful and repeat dose in half an hour. Put a tight binder round the patient's body and bind the legs closely together. Get a doctor or trained nurse as soon as possible, for such bleeding is very dangerous.

POISONS

When the Poison Is Not Known.—When a person has been poisoned and the nature of the poison is unknown, the Emergency Rules are:

1. Send at once for a physician.

2. Empty the stomach with an emetic, such as mustard and salt water.

3. Then give chalk; if necessary, take the plaster from the wall, and mix it with a glass of water. Also three or four raw eggs in a glass of milk.

When a person is unconscious and the cause is unknown, never give alcohol, as the cause may be other than poison, and alcohol on the breath of the person may mislead the physician.

Practice artificial respiration (see article under Reviving the Drowned), and treat as for shock and collapse. (See article on Shock and Collapse.)

When the Poison Is Known.—1. Aconite.—

SYMPTOMS.—The symptoms follow quickly. First come burning and tingling of mouth and lips, followed by numbness. Vomiting occurs in about an hour. The skin is cold and clammy, with a feeling as of ants crawling over the body. The pupils are dilated and the eyes are staring. The pulse is weak and irregular, the gait is staggering and breathing is difficult. Consciousness is present to the end.

TREATMENT.—Make the patient vomit promptly. Apply external heat and give strong black coffee by mouth or rectum. If breathing begins to fail, begin artificial respiration. (See Reviving the Drowned.)

2. Acetanilid, Antipyrin, Phenacetin, Exalgin.—

SYMPTOMS.—Collapse, blueness of skin, slow breathing, weak, irregular pulse, vomiting and profuse sweating.

TREATMENT.—Give hot black coffee and aromatic spirits of ammonia, a teaspoonful in half a glass of water. Apply external heat.

3. Acids—(*Nitric, Oxalic, Sulphuric, Hydrochloric, etc.*).—

SYMPTOMS.—Gastro-intestinal irritation. Burning from mouth to stomach. Corrosion and bleeding of lining of mouth. Difficult swallowing. "Coffee grounds" vomiting. Intense abdominal pain. Shock and collapse.

TREATMENT.—Give soap and water, or lime-water, chalk, or very weak aromatic spirits of ammonia (about a teaspoonful to a glass of water). Follow by milk, white of egg, sweet oil. Give hot coffee by rectum.

4. Alkalies—(*Ammonia, Potash, Lye, Washing Soda, Caustic Soda*).—

SYMPTOMS.—Burning and destruction of lining of mouth. Severe pain, vomiting and shock.

TREATMENT.—Cause vomiting. Vinegar and water in equal parts or the juice of four lemons may be given. Also castor oil and olive oil mixed in equal parts. Treat for shock.

5. Arsenic (*Paris Green, Fowler's Solution, "Rough on Rats"*), Antimony.—

SYMPTOMS.—Faintness, nausea and bloody vomiting. Pain over the stomach. Profuse watery diarrhœa, cramps in leg muscles. Vomiting becomes increasingly violent. Intense thirst. Collapse.

TREATMENT.—Produce vomiting. Give large quantities of dialyzed iron or fresh ferric hydrate, if near a drug store. Give magnesia or large doses of castor oil and water. Stimulate with strong black coffee by mouth or rectum and keep warm.

6. Belladonna, Atropin.—

SYMPTOMS.—The face is flushed, eyes are reddened. Pulse is rapid. Patient is dizzy and walks with staggering gait. Throat is hot and dry. Breathing is slow and deep. Pupils are dilated. Patient is delirious, sometimes wildly so.

TREATMENT.—Produce vomiting. Give coffee enema and aromatic spirits of ammonia by mouth. Use artificial respiration.

7. Carbolic Acid (*Phenol*).—

SYMPTOMS.—When diluted, there are no local symptoms. When concentrated, there is a burning from mouth to stomach. The mouth is white from the corrosion.

Skin is cold and clammy, breathing is slow and

shallow. Patient goes into collapse and unconsciousness.

Treatment.—Give sodium and magnesium sulphate dissolved. If seen immediately after taking, give patient alcohol or else whisky (three tablespoonfuls). Cause vomiting. Give coffee by rectum.

8. Chloral (*Knock-out Drops*).—

Symptoms.—Slow, feeble, irregular pulse, slow breathing and blueness of the face. Skin cold and temperature subnormal. Unconsciousness.

Treatment.—Cause vomiting. Apply external heat and rub the body. Give coffee enemas. Keep patient awake. Use artificial respiration.

9. Cocaine.—

Symptoms.—Pallor, fainting, dizziness and collapse. Heart is weak and breathing slow and shallow.

Treatment.—If the cocaine has been taken by the mouth, give an emetic. Stimulate with whisky and coffee enemas. Use artificial respiration.

Chronic cocainism is impossible to cure except in a sanitarium.

10. Copper (*Blue Vitriol, Verdigris*).—

Symptoms.—Intense corrosion of mouth and stomach, causing pain, bleeding and intestinal cramps.

TREATMENT.—Cause vomiting by mustard water. Then give milk and eggs. Stimulate with black coffee, by rectum, if necessary.

11. Exalgin. ***(See Acetanilid.)*—**

12. Hydrocyanic Acid (*Prussic Acid*).—

SYMPTOMS.—These follow within a second or two after taking. Unconsciousness comes on instantly. Eyes are fixed, pupils dilated, skin cold and clammy and limbs relaxed. Breathing slow, deep and convulsive. Death in a few minutes.

TREATMENT.—Produce vomiting. Give whisky, brandy or strong aromatic spirits of ammonia. Use artificial respiration.

13. Lead. ***Acute and Chronic Poisoning.*—**

(a.) *Acute.*—Symptoms of local irritation. Thirst, vomiting and abdominal colic and constipation. Feeble pulse, quick, shallow breathing, cold, clammy skin and collapse. Convulsions and unconsciousness.

TREATMENT.—Cause vomiting. Give sodium or magnesium sulphate (Epsom Salts) in large doses. Coffee by mouth or rectum and aromatic spirits of ammonia. External warmth.

(b). *Chronic.*—Painters and workers in lead industries are the usual sufferers from this form.

SYMPTOMS.—Blue line on gums. Colic, constipation, anemia. Insanity of a morose nature. Sometimes epilepsy. Inflammation of nerves, showing mainly in wrist drop, a condition in which the hand hangs at the wrist and there is no power to raise it.

TREATMENT.—Discontinue the occupation which exposes to the poisoning. Give Epsom salts every morning to hasten elimination of lead.

14. Mercury (*Corrosive Sublimate, Bichloride of Mercury, Bug Poison*).—

(a.) *Acute.—*

SYMPTOMS.—Severe irritation of stomach and intestines. Great pain, vomiting and diarrhœa. Collapse.

TREATMENT.—Egg albumen, milk. Later, rectal salt water injections.

(b.) *Chronic.—*

SYMPTOMS.—Fetid breath, metallic taste, sore teeth and swollen gums. Excessive saliva. If this continues, the gums bleed, teeth fall out, tongue and mouth ulcerate. There is gradual anemia, wasting, nervous tremors, exhaustion.

TREATMENT.—Discontinue all mercury. Treat the mouth with mild antiseptic mouth washes and give general tonic treatment.

15. Nux Vomica, Strychnine.—

SYMPTOMS.—These come on quickly. There is a sense of suffocation and a panic of apprehension. Then convulsions begin. This is shown first in twitching of the fingers, followed rapidly by convulsions. The body is curved backward from ankles to head. The convulsions are very powerful and cause intense agony. The senses are very acute. Each convulsion lasts a minute or two and is followed by relaxation, sweating and exhaustion. The convulsions increase in severity and frequency. The eyes are staring and fixed; the face shows the "sardonic grin." The jaw muscle is affected last of all, which differentiates the condition from "lockjaw."

TREATMENT.—Cause vomiting. Give large doses of potassium bromide (60 grains) and chloral (30 grains) by rectum. Keep in a dark and absolutely quiet room.

16. Opium (*Morphine*).—

(a.) *Acute.*—

SYMPTOMS.—Drowsiness, sleep, then unconsciousness; the pupils become so small that they are called "pin-point." At first the patient may be aroused; later not. The skin is cold, pulse slow and weak; breathing gradually becomes slower and more irregular.

TREATMENT.—Make the patient vomit. *Keep him awake* by all means. Coffee enemas. Tincture of belladonna, thirty drops by mouth. If in spite of walking, slapping with wet towels, etc., the patient cannot be kept awake, artificial respiration (see Reviving the Drowned) must be resorted to. Keep working for hours as long as the heart continues to beat.

(b.) *Chronic.*—

Symptoms.—This habit is very common. The will power is broken and there is an almost total loss of moral sense. There is gradual loss of weight, anemia and constipation.

Treatment.—All home attempts to cure this habit are unsuccessful except in rare cases. The victim must be put in a sanatorium, where strict watch can be kept over him. He will lie, cheat and steal to obtain the coveted drugs. Few cures are permanent.

17. Phosphorus (*Matches*).—

Symptoms.—*Two stages:*

(a.) Nausea, abdominal pain, vomiting, diarrhœa, collapse. Then gradual recovery for a few days when the second stage begins.

(b.) Jaundice; an enlarged liver, which later shrinks to very small size. There is an intense thirst, bloody vomit and blood in the stools. The pulse is rapid and weak; the skin cold. The urine is scanty and often bloody. Muscular twitchings begin, followed by unconsciousness and death.

Treatment.—Produce vomiting. Give Epsom

salts or citrate of magnesia in large doses and turpentine in 5 to 15 drop doses. If the second stage begins, the case is hopeless.

18. Silver Nitrate.—

SYMPTOMS.—Vomiting of black material, pain, corrosion of mucous membrane of mouth, intestinal colic.

TREATMENT.—Give salt solution (*i. e.*, common salt dissolved in water), to form silver chloride. Then give white of egg and milk.

19. Food or Ptomaine Poisoning.—

This poisoning is caused by food containing bacteria resulting from putrefaction; food infected with disease germs; and food containing parasites. Any meat, fish, shell fish, milk, eggs, cheese, ice cream and canned goods may, under the above conditions, cause ptomaine poisoning.

SYMPTOMS.—In general, the symptoms are vomiting, cramps, diarrhœa, headache, prostration, weak pulse, cold hands and feet, possibly an eruption and shock.

TREATMENT.—Call a physician, and while waiting for him to arrive, rid the patient of the poison by causing repeated vomiting. Water and mustard (one-half a teaspoonful of mustard in a glass of water), or tickling the throat with a finger will cause it. Empty the lower bowel by giving a soap-

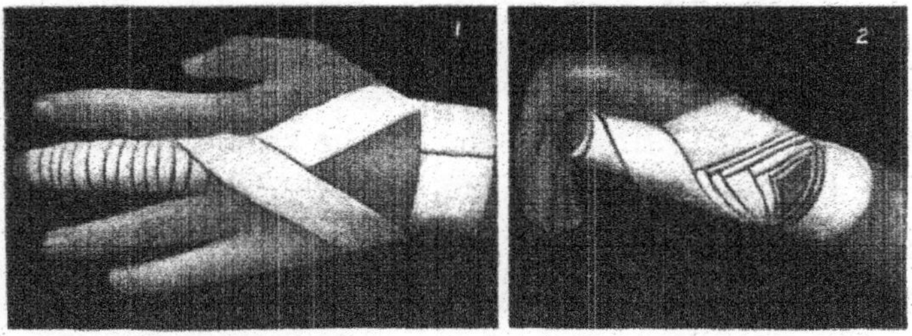

1. SIMPLE ROLLER BANDAGE OF FINGER
2. FIGURE-OF-EIGHT BANDAGE OF THUMB

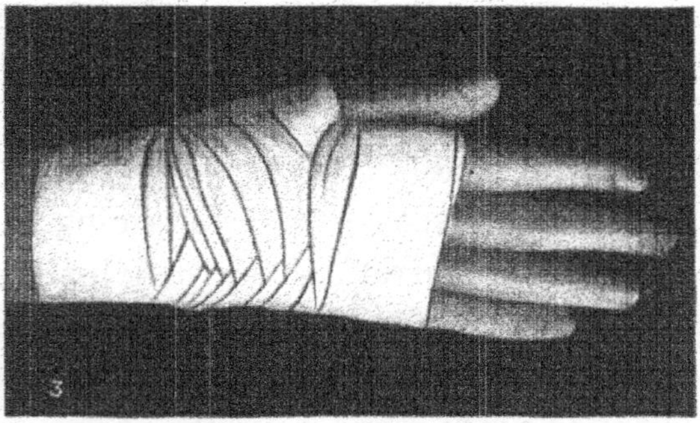

3. FIGURE-OF-EIGHT BANDAGE OF HAND

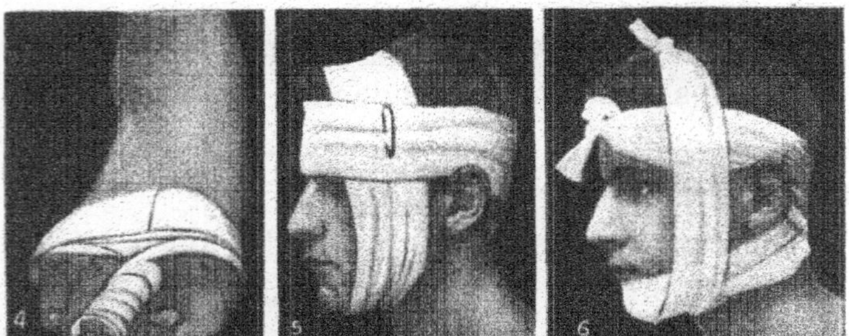

4. ROLLER BANDAGE OF TOE
5. HANDKERCHIEF BANDAGE OF HEAD
6. BANDAGE FOR HOLDING LOWER JAW IN PLACE

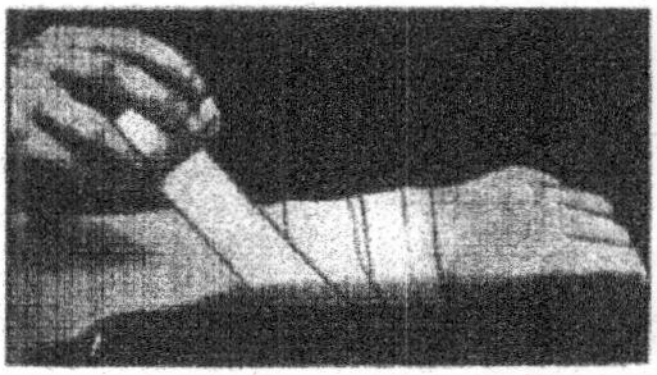

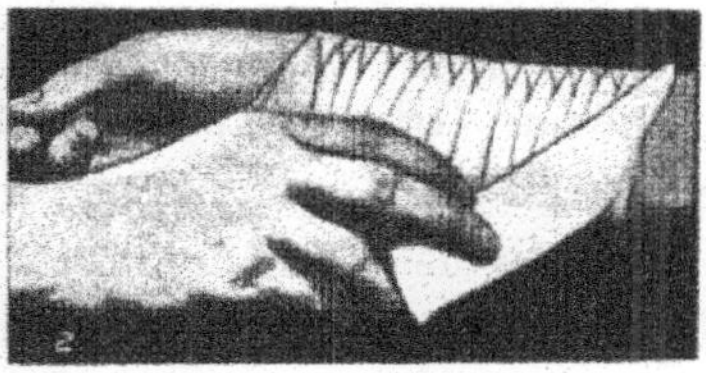

1. BEGINNING A SPIRAL REVERSE BANDAGE OF THE ARM
2. MAKING THE REVERSE TURN. THIS IS DONE AT EVERY OTHER TURN ABOUT THE ARM

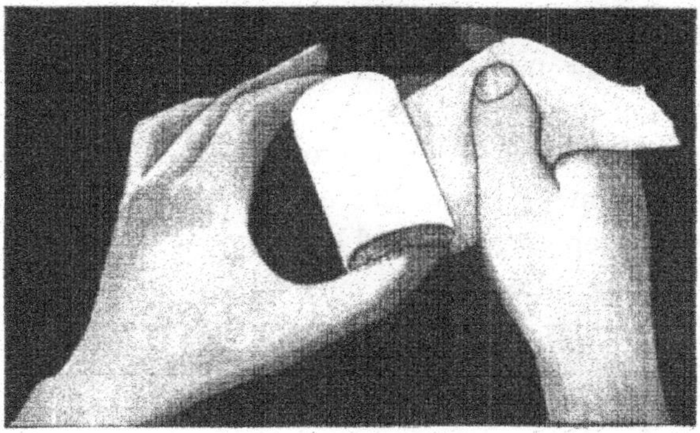

3. HOW TO HOLD A BANDAGE WHEN ROLLING IT

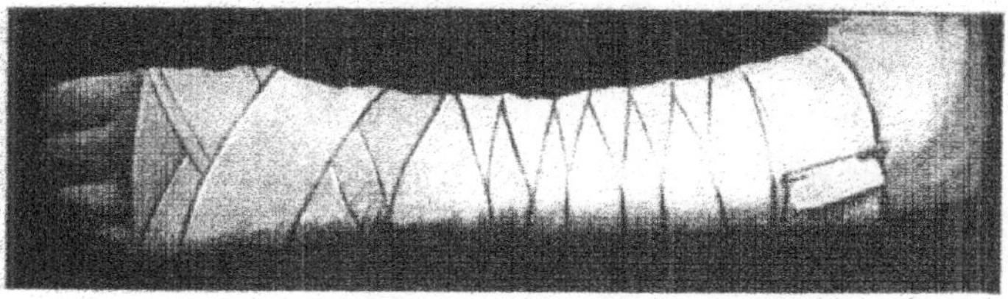

4. BANDAGE OF HAND AND ARM WHEN FINISHED

suds enema. (See chapter on Home Nursing.) Support the heart and nerve force with a tablespoonful of whisky and hot water every half hour, or oftener as needed. Put hot water bottles at the feet and keep the body warm with blankets.

BITES AND STINGS

Mosquitoes.—It is the female mosquito which is harmful. Either during or after sucking blood, she injects a poisonous matter into the body. This causes itching, swelling, and in some people an inflammation of the skin.

Malaria and yellow fever are transmitted by certain forms of mosquitoes. In tropical countries, all living and sleeping rooms and beds should have mosquito netting. People live only a very short time in the tropics before they are enlightened concerning the mosquito and her habits.

This is no place to discuss the various species of mosquitoes. Suffice it to say that one is called the Culex, the other Anopheles. The latter communicates malaria.

The Culex lays her eggs in sinks, tanks, cisterns and water about houses, while the Anopheles deposits hers in shallow pools and sluggish streams, especially those on which there is a growth of vegetation commonly called "green scum."

All pools, ponds and marshy districts should be drained, and in the malarial season petroleum poured on the surface, to destroy the eggs of the mosquito. (See chapter on Fevers.)

TREATMENT.—Put the hands in a one per cent. solution of carbolic acid, and while they are wet rub them on all exposed surfaces. A combination of kerosene and water will have the same effect.

After having been bitten by a mosquito, an alkali of some sort, as ammonia water or baking soda in water, applied to the affected parts on cloths, is beneficial. As an emergency measure, clay and water or a mud poultice may be used.

Bee, Wasp and Hornet Sting.—The bee stings but once, as the sting breaks off and is retained in the flesh of the victim. A wasp or hornet can repeat the act. It is well to extract the sting of bees immediately.

Ammonia is the best remedy for relieving pain.

Snake and Spider Bite.—It is beyond the scope of this book to go into details regarding the different snake and spider bites.

SYMPTOMS.—The symptoms of snake and spider bites of all poisonous species are similar.

1. Some pain in the wound.
2. Swelling and redness of part. Pain increases.

3. Discoloration of the part bitten, sometimes followed by gangrene.

4. Vital centres of brain controlling the heart and breathing apparatus are slowly paralyzed by the poison.

5. Often drowsiness and stupor.

6. Breathing is labored.

7. Pulse weak and irregular.

8. Shock.

TREATMENT.—Make the wound bleed as much as possible. Keep the poison out of the general blood stream by applying a tourniquet above and below wound. Cut out, by oval cuts on each side, the flesh below and around the wound.

Pour potassium permanganate solution into the wound.

For weak heart give whisky, in large doses, until recovery ensues.

If you are going to a section inhabited by venomous snakes or spiders you should inject yourself with a dose of Calmette's anti-venomous serum every two or three weeks. This is a preventive. If this serum is used, do not use whisky.

Sucking the wound is generally of little use.

Get a physician as soon as possible.

Dog and Cat Bite.—If you live in a city, go at once to a hospital or to a physician; otherwise, observe the following rules for dog and cat bite:

1. Find out whether or not the animal is mad. If it is, send the patient to the Pasteur Institute, New York City, or to the nearest municipal Board of Health.

2. To get the poison from wound, encourage bleeding.

3. Cauterize with red hot nail or poker.

4. A solution of carbolic acid (a teaspoonful in a pint of water), poured into the wound is good. Bandage the wound with clean dressings.

CHAPTER IV

DISEASES OF THE SKIN

THERE are many diseases of the skin for which the layman can do nothing but consult a doctor immediately. But there are some of the more common ailments which he can easily understand and alleviate. In general, it may be said that all skin diseases have a rash or eruption, and all rashes cause itching. If this rash or eruption is accompanied by fever, vomiting, headache and general sick feeling, it is very probable that some specific disease is present and a doctor should be sent for promptly. It is well, at the same time, to isolate the patient, especially if it is a child, and there are other children in the family.

Itching (*Pruritus*).—This is not a disease, but a symptom. It occurs in most diseases of the skin, and in some general diseases, such as gout and diabetes, an intense itching may be felt. To cure the itching permanently, of course the disease must be cured, but the suffering of intense itching is so great that means must be used to stop the trouble temporarily. The following are a few remedies which may be safely tried until the doctor can see the patient.

TREATMENT.—1. For itching over large surface, general baths are excellent. Cold or tepid baths are best. Add to the bath one or two pounds of baking soda, or bran water, made by boiling bran, tied in a bag, in water. After the bath, powder the body with talcum, boric acid powder or even powdered starch.

2. For itching over small areas, bathe the parts with any of the following:

(a.) Baking soda, teaspoonful to pint of water.

(b.) Equal parts of alcohol and water.

(c.) Equal parts of vinegar and water.

(d.) Calamine lotion. (See Appendix.)

3. For scaly, dry eruptions with itching, an ointment is better, but this should be prescribed by a doctor, as different diseases require quite different treatment. For temporary use, vaseline or Lassar's Paste is good.

CHAFING AND CHAPPING

Chafing is caused by two skin surfaces rubbing together when those surfaces are irritated by sweat or other discharge. This usually occurs in hot weather, after exercise, or when clothing rubs against the skin. The part chafed is red, hot and tender.

Chapping is the term usually applied to a condition of the lips, which occurs in very cold weather and when saliva is allowed to run over the lips freely. The sensitive mucous membrane cracks and peels off. The process is essentially the same as that of chafing.

TREATMENT.—First of all, remove cause if it is due to any discharge. Then clean parts thoroughly. Keep talcum powder or boric acid powder on parts constantly. If the lips are dry and peeling, vaseline or cold cream will be better than the powder.

Pimples, Blackheads (*Acne*).—This eruption appears on the face, head and shoulders. Usually it comes at the age of puberty in both boys and girls and continues through adolescence. It consists of a conical elevation of the skin, usually red and tender, which is called a pimple. These pimples form into little pustules, discharging matter after a few days, or else they become blackheads. These are small black spots in the skin which can be squeezed out in little worm-like masses. They are due to an inflammation of the oil glands of the skin. The end of the gland becomes clogged and blackened, presenting the appearance known as "blackhead." If an infection occurs, a pimple follows. This condition is very unsightly in young people and results sometimes in permanent scars, so that it is important to begin treatment at once. This condition indicates a general low state of health. Chronic constipation and anemia accompany this condition. Frequently, habits of eating, the kind of food eaten, lack of fresh air and neglect of exercise are contributing causes.

TREATMENT.—The general treatment is by far the most important. The boy or girl should be made to take plenty of outdoor exercise, plenty of sleep and good plain food. Eating between meals should be forbidden, and all rich food, as well as tea and coffee, prohibited. If the child is pale and anemic the doctor should prescribe some suitable tonic. The daily movement of the bowels should be carefully attended to. Cold baths or daily warm baths, with vigorous scrubbing and rubbing of the body and face, are very helpful.

Local treatment consists in keeping the skin clean and well toned up by bathing in hot water and Castile soap, followed by cold water immediately after. All pimples, when they have matter in them, should be opened by pressure and the pus discharged. Blackheads should be squeezed out, taking care not to bruise the skin too much. Calamine lotion (see Appendix) is good to put on the face at night after bathing it. But, in general, for any medicinal ointment or lotion a patient must apply to a doctor, who can see the condition and understand it.

Eczema, Salt Rheum, Tetter.—Eczema is believed by many pathologists to be a catarrhal inflammation of the skin. The exudate (fluid that escapes) is beneath the surface until the top is scratched away. There are two general varieties.

1. Eczema of internal origin, due to some disturbance of feeding or nutrition, or to some drug.
2. Eczema of external origin. This is caused by occupation or occasionally by climate.

TREATMENT.—The internal eczema usually occurs symmetrically on both sides of the body. Both cheeks, both arms, or both feet are affected. To cure this, the general treatment is most important. The patient must have his bowels in proper condition, diet must be carefully regulated, usually all meat and rich pastry being avoided. The local treatment need only be to allay itching and infection.

External eczema, on the contrary, needs simply local treatment. First of all, stop using the particular fluid or substance which irritates the skin.

This alone will heal most eczemas, if the affected part is not scratched and irritated.

For a "weeping" or exuding surface, use a lotion such as calamine lotion. Do not use water on eczema except once a day with soap to clean off crusts and scales. If the eczema is old and thickened, an irritating ointment to stimulate it is indicated. But for these a doctor's advice is necessary.

Baldness and Dandruff.—Baldness is usually accompanied by dandruff, and is thought to be caused by it. Dandruff is an inflammation of the scalp, with the formation of greasy, yellowish-white flakes or scales. Its correct name is *Seborrhœa* of the scalp. The wearing of tight, hard hats by men is undoubtedly a factor in the large percentage of bald heads among young men.

First remove the scales by rubbing in vaseline or sweet oil and then shampoo with green soap. After this, rub into scalp an alcoholic solution of *resorcin,* 2 per cent. in strength. This latter should be done every night. The shampooing should not be oftener than every two or three weeks.

Hives, Nettle Rash (*Urticaria*).—Urticaria is an acute inflammation of the skin, characterized by the sudden appearance of oval lumps on the skin, white, with an area surrounding it of red or deep pink. There is great itching and burning.

These lumps appear and disappear. Scratching is usually continued until the surface is removed, leaving a raw spot. This relieves the intolerable itch. The whole attack usually lasts only a few days. Very rarely it occurs in the throat and may cause suffocation.

Eating some particular food, such as strawberries or other acid fruits, lobster or other shell fish, frequently causes an attack. The handling of nettles or jellyfish may also produce it. In some people the bites of mosquitoes and fleas will produce urticaria.

TREATMENT.—Avoid eating the food which causes the trouble and take a good cathartic. Locally, a solution of baking soda or vinegar and water, equal parts, is very good. Calamine lotion can also be used. At the first signs of choking, send for a doctor. In the meantime give patient something to make him vomit, as *e. g.* a half-teaspoonful of mustard in half a pint of warm water, to be swallowed quickly.

Cold Sore, Fever Blister.—These usually appear on the lips, although they may occur anywhere on the face. Cold sores consist of groups of little raised blisters. There may be several of these groups. There is a good deal of itching and burning, but disfigurement is the greatest annoyance.

Cold sores usually result from indigestion, or from the irritation of the nasal discharge accompanying cold in the head.

Treatment.—Apply spirits of camphor in early stages. Later, to allay the itching and burning, apply calamine lotion. (See Appendix.)

Ringworm.—This is a contagious skin disease caused by a fungus. It appears as a small, red, scaly spot, the edge of which shows small scaly pimples. As the circle gets bigger, the centre heals. Ringworm of the scalp occurs as a circular scaly patch, grayish red with stubs of hair sticking out. These are easily pulled out. A doctor must be consulted to treat ringworm, as it is not easily cured. Until a doctor is called, however, painting the ringworm with pure tincture of iodine is very good treatment.

Prickly Heat.—This is a fine red rash which breaks out on children and adults in hot weather. Copious sweating and a congestion of the sweat glands cause this rash.

Treatment.—Keep the body well bathed in cold water and weak alcohol. Then apply talcum or boric acid powder. If the itching is excessive a saturated solution of baking soda will relieve it.

Ivy Poison.—Certain plants—poison ivy, poison sumach and poison oak—cause an acute inflammatory condition of the skin. In some people this is so severe that the patient is really ill, with fever and sometimes delirium.

TREATMENT.—After being exposed to the poison ivy a thorough bathing with soap and water will remove most of the pollen which causes the eruption. After the eruption appears, apply a saturated solution of baking soda or a solution of vinegar and borax (a teaspoonful of borax to a glass of vinegar). Aristol powder rubbed in is very good. After the eruption appears, avoid water until the acute stage of the rash is past.

Warts.—These are round or flattened projections on the skin. They are not painful unless injured. In children they appear and disappear without apparent cause. If their location or number is annoying they may be burned away with a caustic stick or by painting with chromic acid. In older people the presence of warts is more serious and sometimes is a forerunner of malignant disease—cancer or sarcoma.

Corns and Callus.—These are both thickenings of the skin. The corn is a small circumscribed thickening, while the callous is a more general thickening. Poorly fitting shoes are the main cause of corns. The best cure is, therefore, to wear properly fitting shoes.

TREATMENT.—To remove a corn, soften it with hot water and soap and then carefully cut it away. A solution of salicylic acid, 20 grains to half an ounce of flexible collodion, painted on daily, will remove the corn, leaving a sensitive spot that must be protected for a few days.

Lice (*Pediculi*).—There are three varieties of these: Head lice, clothes lice and the "crab" lice, which inhabit the hair, especially about the sexual organs, from which they spread to other parts of the body.

The head lice, as their name indicates, live on the head and lay their eggs on the hairs. These eggs, or "nits," are little white bodies stuck fast to the hair. They usually hatch out in about six days.

Lice produce intense itching of the scalp. The scratching causes an inflammation and the raw spots become infected. This infection is carried to the glands of the back of the neck, which become enlarged and tender. Lice are very common among dirty, careless people, but they also occur among the cleanest, owing to accidental contact with people who are infested.

TREATMENT.—In children, the hair should be cut short if possible. The hair and scalp should be thoroughly washed with soap. The best household remedy is kerosene and olive oil, equal parts, rubbed into the hair and allowed to stay there overnight. In the morning, wash the hair with hot water and soap and comb out with a fine comb. The "nits" can only be dissolved off with vinegar or alcohol. Instead of kerosene, tincture of larkspur may be rubbed into the hair.

Clothes lice always live in the clothes of filthy people and only come out on the body to feed.

TREATMENT.—Destroy the infected clothes; then keep the body and clothes clean.

The "crab" louse looks very much like a tiny crab. It inhabits the hair and skin surrounding the sexual organs. Itching and scratching call attention to these parasites. Kerosene or blue ointment (10 per cent.) rubbed in will destroy these pests, but the treatment must be repeated several times, at intervals of a week, to insure complete destruction of all eggs.

Scabies (*The Itch*).—This is a skin disease which occurs in all classes of people, although the dirty are most commonly affected. It is due to a small parasite which burrows in the skin. This causes an intense itching, especially at night, when the parasite crawls out of its burrow. The usual places for the eruption of scabies are between the fingers, across the chest and between the shoulders; also around the waist where the clothes restrict.

TREATMENT.—Sulphur is the best drug to kill the parasite. It may be applied as an ointment (10 per cent.). This is rubbed on the body; the patient puts over it some old thick underclothes and sleeps in them. In the morning he takes a bath. This is repeated for three nights, and then the patient discontinues treatment for three or four days. Then repeat the process.

A cleaner but slower way is to scatter between the sheets a couple of tablespoonfuls of powdered flowers of sulphur. The heat of the body volatilizes the sulphur and it is absorbed, but more slowly. A cure with this method takes at least two or three weeks.

CHAPTER V

DISEASES OF THE RESPIRATORY SYSTEM

General Symptoms.—Dyspnœa is the term used to denote difficult breathing. Dyspnœa may be caused by an obstruction of the air passages, by pressure on any part of the respiratory system from without, by tumors or distention of the abdomen, by diseases of the lungs and the covering of the lungs, called the pleura; by heart disease, asthma, anemia, paralysis of the muscles of respiration as the result of bleeding, brain troubles and poisonous agents in the blood.

When a person has difficult breathing or is short of breath, with no previous violent exertion, the condition is a serious one, peculiar to lung or heart disease, and a doctor's advice is needed.

Cough may be caused by direct irritation as the result of breathing irritant vapors or dust, or the presence of foreign bodies; but, as a rule, it is due to an inflammation of either the pharynx, larynx, trachea, bronchi. or lungs. It may also be caused by a reflex irritation. When there is a cough without expectoration it is called a Dry Cough. With expectoration it is known as a Moist Cough. A cough having a metallic, ringing sound, is called a laryngeal or croupy cough.

Sputum is a general name for all material coughed up from the lungs.

Sputum that is either watery or serous, mucopurulent or offensive in odor, or purulent (consisting entirely of pus or "matter"); sputum that occurs in round, flat disks which sink when placed in water; fetid sputum which, when left standing, separates into three distinct layers; rusty sputum, or reddish-brown sputum—all show that disease is present and a physician should be consulted in order to determine the gravity of the condition.

DISEASES OF THE LARYNX

Acute Catarrhal Laryngitis (*Hoarseness*).—The attack begins rather suddenly, with a feeling of dryness, rawness or tickling of the throat. There is hoarseness and attempts are made to cough. Swallowing causes pain. The membrane of the throat is swollen and secretions are diminished. Attempts at talking cause more or less pain in the throat. After a day or two there is a slight expectoration, and then, in a short time, this is increased and there is a loose cough. There may be a slight fever.

Tonsilitis.—The attack begins with fever, white-coated tongue, hot skin and flushed face, hoarse and whispering voice, hard, croupy cough, and (with children) great restlessness. At night time there may be attacks of suffocation.

TREATMENT.—Simple sore throat is not necessarily alarming, but the possibilities are so serious that medical advice should be secured upon the appearance of severe symptoms. As a rule, the patient is well in a week, but in severe cases recovery may take from two to three weeks. The patient should be kept in a room of even temperature, the air kept moist by the vapor of boiling water. Trying to talk should be stopped. Hot mustard foot baths are good. The bowels should be moved freely by either salts or calomel, one grain in ten doses of a tenth of a grain each. Inhalations are both soothing and curative. A very good inhalation is made by putting one or two teaspoonfuls of the compound tincture of benzoin in a quart of boiling water and inhaling the vapor hourly. A weak mustard plaster on the neck, followed by wrapping hot cloths about the neck, may afford relief.

If choking occurs, call a doctor immediately.

Edematous Laryngitis (*Edema of the Glottis*). —Edema is a condition of swelling in which the tissues are filled with a watery fluid.

Edema of the glottis is a swelling of the vocal chords, which partly closes the aperture through which we breathe. The beginning of the trouble is the same as in simple sore throat, but the symptoms gradually get worse. There is a feeling as of a foreign body in the throat, and breathing becomes difficult. Swallowing is difficult. The voice becomes almost lost. The cough becomes suppressed. There is no expectoration, and only after great effort is a little frothy mucus raised. Breathing causes a whistling sound. The patient sits up in bed, mouth open, gasping for breath, with protruding eyes, and the whole body trembling with intense convulsive movements. After a time the face assumes a bluish tinge. Then all these symptoms subside, and in a short while the attack begins again. Unless nature or treatment affords prompt relief, death very often occurs from asphyxia.

Treatment.—Early and vigorous treatment is the only hope of recovery. Put leeches over the throat. Give the patient ice-pellets to hold in the back of the throat until dissolved. In all cases give food and stimulants by the rectum. (See chapter on Home Nursing.) Above all, call a physician with all possible speed.

Croup, Spasmodic Laryngitis.—This is a catarrhal inflammation of the membrane of the larynx, associated with temporary spasmodic contraction of the glottis; characterized by paroxysmal coughing, difficult breathing and attacks of threatening suffocation.

It is caused by changes in climate, "taking cold," excesses in eating and drinking and violent excitement.

As a rule, the attack begins at night time, the child going to bed in apparent health or with a slight fever. After sleeping a few hours it is suddenly awakened by severe coughing, which is dry and ringing, and by a suffocating sensation. After from a half hour to two hours the breathing becomes easier; the cough is not so croupy, the skin becomes covered with more or less of a sweat and the child falls asleep. There will be a loose cough present the next day. Unless treated, the same condition will happen the next night, only not so severely, and again the following nights, each time lessening in severity until the disease disappears entirely.

TREATMENT.—Simple croup always ends favorably. During the attack, place the child in a hot bath. Hot or cold cloths should be wrapped about the throat. At the same time dissolve a teaspoonful of bicarbonate of soda in a glass of water and give a teaspoonful every fifteen minutes until relief is obtained. After the attack, give the child a grain of calomel, and follow it in six or eight hours with a dose of castor oil or magnesia.

DISEASES OF THE BRONCHIAL TUBES

Acute Bronchitis (***Cold on the Chest***).—The condition is very common in children, especially during the teething time. In old age it often occurs again. It often accompanies infectious fevers, such as typhoid fever, influenza, whooping-cough and measles.

There is fever, pain in the chest, a feeling of constriction of the chest, hard breathing, and an expectoration, scanty at first, but soon becoming profuse in amount.

Constipation may be present. A feeling of depression is often experienced.

Recovery of the patient is the rule.

Treatment.—The patient should be kept in a well-ventilated room, and, if a very young child or very aged person, in bed. Give from one-half to two grains of calomel in doses of one-tenth of a grain every fifteen minutes, and follow this in six hours with Epsom salts. A mustard foot-bath will be found beneficial.

Chronic Bronchitis (***Winter Cough***).—This often results from repeated attacks of "cold on the chest," or it may be due to exposure to cold and wet. It is common in old people, and may accompany many other conditions.

The cough, which may not be present, is usually worse at night and early in the morning. It may disappear and return, continuing in this manner for years. The expectoration is usually more or less profuse.

Treatment.—See a physician. Keep the patient warm, but give him fresh air. This disease is often checked or even completely cured by a change of climate—sometimes to a warmer, sometimes to a colder. The advice of a physician is imperatively necessary.

Asthma.—Asthma is characterized by spasmodic attacks of distressing expiratory dyspnœa. The attack may continue a few hours, days or weeks. Men are more subject to it than women.

The first attack of asthma is abrupt. The other attacks throw out premonitory signals which the patient soon learns to know. They are: Watery eyes, irritation in the throat, feeling of constriction of the chest, marked dyspepsia, or the scanty passage of pale urine.

In most cases the attack begins in the early hours of morning or during the afternoon with a feeling of fear, a binding of the chest and a great desire for air. The breathing becomes a loud wheeze, the face becomes red, or it may become blue, and be bathed in perspiration. The eyeballs may protrude and the neck muscles become prominent, as they aid in the fight for air. The difficulty in breathing soon becomes so severe that the patient feels as if death is near at hand. After some minutes or hours the breathing becomes easier, the symptoms abate and the attack gradually ceases. The patient is exhausted and has a loose cough.

Asthma is a chronic affection and permanent recovery is rare. The attacks may be relieved by treatment. Asthma itself does not cause death, but it may cause injury to vital organs which may terminate fatally.

Treatment.—A physician should be called and he may instruct the patient how to meet future attacks. Relief is sometimes obtained from drinking strong black coffee. If taken in time, coffee may even ward off an impending attack. But common sense demands the advice of a doctor.

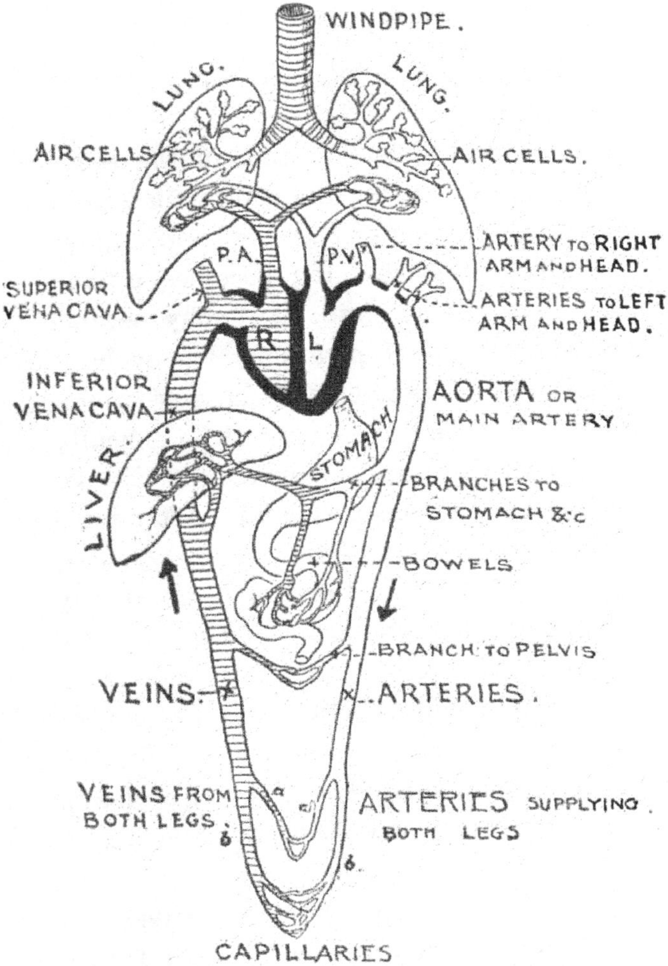

DIAGRAM, SHOWING COMPLETE CIRCULATORY SYSTEM

It may be mentioned that exercise, almost to the fatiguing point, bathing, regulated diet, and, if possible, a change of climate, are wonderfully beneficial.

Hay-Asthma (*Hay Fever, Rose Cold*).—This condition most commonly occurs during the Summer and Autumn. In many cases the condition of the nervous system is a predisposing cause. There are other causes, such as heredity, sedentary life, nasal disease, and especially the inhalation of irritating dusts or vapors, or the pollen of grasses, rye, corn, wheat or roses.

Symptoms.—An attack of hay fever begins with irritation of the eyes, which become watery; the nose runs, and the patient sneezes a clear, watery discharge. The congestion extends down the throat, causing a croupy, wheezing cough. The breathing becomes difficult, and may resemble that of asthma.

The attacks end after a few days and may begin again after a few days or weeks, to remit and then begin again, and so on until the season is over.

Hay asthma is never fatal, but true asthma, chronic bronchitis or the loss of the sense of hearing or the sense of smell may result.

Treatment.—This disease has no specific. There is no drug that will cure.

Consult a physician, who will determine whether or not any nasal trouble is present. Often a slight operation will be followed by a cure of hay fever.

Often a change of climate will prevent an attack of hay asthma. A sea voyage is good, and many find relief in certain elevated regions. The general health should be closely watched. As a rule, the patient is more or less run down and requires tonics.

Cases of indigestion should receive prompt attention. Avoid constipation by taking calomel in doses of one-tenth of a grain for ten doses and following it six hours later with salts, such as a half ounce of Epsom salts in water.

The diet should be made up of fruits and vegetables for the most part, and animal foods, coffee and tea should be interdicted. Frequent hot baths should be the rule. To abort the attack, five grains of quinine, three times a day, given one month before the attack is expected have often proved successful.

There are many nasal sprays that are beneficial, but see a doctor about a prescription for a spray and do not use advertised hay fever spraying medicines, for these have for their main ingredient cocaine, the use of which has produced numberless drug fiends.

Pulmonary Hemorrhage, Hemoptysis, Hemorrhage from Lungs.—Pulmonary hemorrhage is the spitting of pure or unmixed blood, which is usually of a bright red color and follows the act of coughing. "Spitting of blood" occurs suddenly; in a few cases it is preceded by nose bleed, palpitation of the heart and difficult breathing.

The patient feels a tickling sensation in the throat, followed by a salty taste in the mouth; he coughs to remove it, and warm, red, frothy blood rushes from the mouth and nose. Naturally, the sight of so much blood frightens the patient. He becomes depressed, pale, nervous, and often faints. The attack may last a half hour or it may last several hours, returning for several days, and in the meantime the expectoration may be either bloody or streaked with blood. Following the bleeding there is a slight fever and pain in the chest.

Bleeding from the lungs may be distinguished from "nose bleed," by the fact that in bleeding from the lungs the blood is frothy and bright red; from stomach bleeding, by the fact that blood from the stomach is dark red in color and usually mixed with the contents of the stomach. In certain cases the blood may come from the lungs and get into the stomach and then be vomited, but in these cases the raising of blood is preceded by pain in the stomach.

Pulmonary hemorrhage, in itself, rarely ends fatally, except in advanced cases of "consumption," and although it causes severe collapse, the patient recovers rapidly, unless pneumonia follows.

TREATMENT.—Assure the patient there is no danger, put him to bed, with head and shoulders elevated and require absolute quiet. Cold drinks and small pieces of ice may be given. Unless it causes chilliness, an ice bag on the chest may be of value. Common table salt slowly dissolved in the mouth is a very popular remedy, and while of little or no benefit, serves to occupy the attention of the patient until medical advice is obtained, which should be at the earliest possible opportunity. (See Consumption.)

DISEASES OF THE LUNGS

In discussing diseases of the lungs, only the signs which every one notices will be considered. The purpose is to have the early symptoms appreciated, in order that a doctor may be called in time to be of some service. In most cases it is beyond the power of the ordinary individual to do more than make the patient comfortable.

Pneumonia.—The affection begins with a severe and usually prolonged chill, followed by a high fever. In children, convulsions often take the place of the chill, and sometimes, in adults, there is vomiting instead of the chill.

From the beginning of the disease the collapse and prostration are decided. There may be distressing feelings in the chest, made worse by coughing; breathing becomes difficult. The face becomes flushed and the cheek bones assume a peculiar mahogany blush. Palpitation of the heart may be present. The cough is dry at first, followed by scanty, frothy expectorations, slightly streaked with blood. The lips become more or less blue and sores develop upon them. Combined with these symptoms there may be nose bleed, headache, sleeplessness and stomach disturbances. Delirium may be present, and is a grave sign. If the patient has been a hard drinker, the outcome of the disease is doubtful.

What to do While Waiting for the Doctor.—Put the patient to bed in a light, well-aired room, avoiding drafts, but keeping windows open. Remove all clothing. An undershirt is entirely unnecessary, and light bed covers are the best. The diet should be of the most nutritious kind, but easily digestible in character, and should be given at short intervals, as once every three hours. Strong black coffee is good for the patient, as are chicken broths and milk. If the tongue is coated and the stomach in bad condition, calomel in one-quarter of a grain doses for eight doses, followed in two hours after the last dose by a mild dose of salts, is recommended.

Poultices are of little value, but home-made mustard plasters, applied to the chest, may be used. (See chapter on Home Nursing.)

If the fever is high, sponging with alcohol and cold water, or even cold water alone, will give relief.

Tuberculosis (*Consumption*).—Consumption is caused by a germ. A person cannot have consumption without the germ; but the germ may be inhaled and yet the person not have consumption.

If a person living in a cold, damp tenement, breathing dust and noxious vapors, with exhausted vitality, inhales the germ he is liable to have consumption. Almost any disease of the lungs prepares the way for consumption.

There is a form of the disease called "Galloping Consumption." A person is attacked suddenly, wastes away and dies in a comparatively short time. The signs of this form of consumption are rapid loss of weight, high fever, night sweats, hurried breathing, pains in the chest, cough, profuse expectoration and rapid prostration.

This disease is most frequent between the ages of puberty and middle life.

Consumption, as commonly observed, begins slowly and steals on the individual insidiously. The symptoms are loss of appetite, dyspepsia, and distress in the stomach after meals. The sufferer becomes pallid, anemic and notices that he has lost a little weight and feels weaker than when he was in good health. All these symptoms may easily mislead both the patient and physician.

Later in the progress of the disease, he has a slight, dry, hacking cough, usually in the morning, with a scanty, glairy expectoration. He loses more weight, he notices that his heart becomes irritable, and he has a pain in his chest, most marked below the shoulder blades. He may have a hemorrhage from the lungs, either slight or very profuse. Slight "colds" tend to aggravate all these manifestations.

When the condition is well advanced, the cough becomes worse, the expectoration may be green in color; there are night sweats, and evening fever and shortness of breath increase. The eyes are very bright, the face is flushed, and a sensation of burning of the soles and palms is present. A chronic diarrhœa may be present. Bleeding from the lungs may occur any time, but it is most frequent and profuse during the last stages. The emaciation, pallor and weakness become extreme. The mind remains clear and the victims are hopeful to the very last.

TREATMENT.—*To prevent the spread of Consumption,* a person with the disease should expectorate in a vessel containing a solution of bichloride of mercury, carbolic acid solution, or caustic alkalies. Otherwise, the sputum dries and is rapidly disseminated throughout the atmosphere, where it may be inhaled by persons prepared to contract the disease. Paper napkins, pasteboard spit-cups, rags and other inexpensive materials may be used to receive the expectoration also, which (a great advantage) may be destroyed by burning. In most cities there is a law prohibiting spitting on the floor of public buildings, cars and thoroughfares. Draperies not needed and unnecessary upholstery that cannot be easily cleansed, should be removed from the living rooms of tuberculous patients. All foods should be well cooked if "consumption" is suspected. Living in low, damp places should be avoided by a consumptive or a person susceptible to the disease. Fresh air, sunshine and outdoor life are of vital importance. A high altitude, where the air is dry and rare, and the climate equable, is best for most patients. Bathing, cold sponging, nutritious diet and moderation in eating and drinking should be prescribed.

As to Climates.—Colorado and New Mexico are types of high, cold and dry climates, while inland Southern California may be taken to represent a warm, dry climate. Warm and moist climates are to be found on the coast of Southern California and in Florida. If it is impossible to move a patient to these places, a nearby country place among the hills, away from damp regions, where plenty of fresh air and sunshine can be enjoyed, will serve the purpose nearly as well. The city is no place for a consumptive. The hygienic treatment is important. The living rooms of a consumptive should be so situated as to be open to air and sunlight as many hours of the day as possible. The atmosphere should not be too dry, as cough and subsequent hemorrhage may be caused thereby. The temperature should average 65° F. It is best that the bedroom be occupied only at night and well aired during the day. The clothing should be warm and loose, and thin woolen or loosely woven cotton underwear should be worn throughout the year. A daily bath, followed by a vigorous rubbing, is recommended. Cold sea bathing is harmful. Exhaustion should be avoided. The presence of fever is always a signal for rest. Avoid sedentary occupations and indulge in quiet but frequent amusement.

Nutritious food, such as meats, poultry, game, oysters, fish, animal broths, milk, eggs, etc., are always beneficial. Nothing, however, should be fried. Avoid such foods as pork, veal, hot bread, cakes, pies, pastry, sweetmeats, rich gravies, crabs, lobsters, etc.

Water in liberal quantities is beneficial. Cod liver oil taken just before meals is helpful.

We do not discuss the medical treatment, as in this age of enlightenment, with tuberculosis exhibits everywhere and societies in every section to instruct the community regarding tuberculosis, the average individual knows enough to seek medical aid promptly, and obtain a correct diagnosis.

Pleurisy (*Stitch in the Side*).—The lungs are invested, upon the exterior surface, with an exceedingly delicate serous membrane, the pleura. This membrane becomes inflamed, from several causes, and pleurisy results.

The acute variety of pleurisy usually starts with a chill, which is followed in a short time by a sharp, shooting pain, usually near the right nipple or in the armpit. Coughing and breathing make it worse. The breathing is rapid, and a dry, short, hacking cough is present, with a slight fever. If fluid forms, the pain lessens, the shortness of the breath grows worse, blueness of the face develops, the cough becomes very distressing and the patient assumes a look of anxiety.

There is a form of pleurisy which begins slowly, usually after cold, exposure and fatigue. The individual first complains of a sense of weariness, shortness of the breath, which becomes worse on slight exertion, fever at night time, followed by sweats, a short cough, but little or no expectoration, and a "stitch" in the side.

Treatment.—The patient should be put to bed at once and should lie on the affected side. By doing this, the chest movements on that side while breathing are lessened and the pain will not be so severe. The diet should be of a liquid or semi-solid nature. When the condition is first noticed, give two grains of calomel in doses of a quarter of a grain every fifteen minutes, and six hours after the last dose administer a half an ounce of magnesium sulphate. A physician should be called instantly to care for a case of pleurisy, because of its dangerous character and rapid progress.

CHAPTER VI

DISEASES OF THE DIGESTIVE SYSTEM

DISEASES OF THE STOMACH

Acute Indigestion, Acute Gastritis or Bilious Fever.—Acute indigestion is an acute catarrhal inflammation of the mucous membrane of the stomach, caused by the presence of foods that are indigestible, by the drinking of alcoholic beverages to excess, or by certain irritating medicines, corrosive poisons, exposure to cold and wet, and infectious fevers.

SYMPTOMS.—Usually there is a loss of appetite, the tongue is heavily coated and the breath has a bad odor. Nausea is present and there may sometimes be vomiting. A slight fever accompanies the condition, with headache, flashes of heat, and sensations of burning in the palms of the hands. The abdomen is tender, and the patient has a distressed feeling and pains in the stomach.

Eructations of wind are common; there may be fainting spells and either constipation or diarrhœa. At the end of the attack there may be little sores about the lips and mouth.

As a rule, the duration of a mild case of acute indigestion is one week.

TREATMENT.—The stomach must have a rest. If vomiting occurs and the stomach is overloaded with food, give copious draughts of hot water. It is important to cleanse the bowels thoroughly.

Calomel in a dose of from five to ten grains, combined with five grains of bicarbonate of soda and followed in about six hours with an ounce of magnesium sulphate or a full dose of some mineral water will speedily cause the stomach to regain its tone. The calomel, however, should be given in divided doses every fifteen minutes of either a tenth or a quarter of a grain. After the stomach and bowels have been emptied, eating may be resumed. But only the most bland (easily digested) food should be given at first. Medical aid should be obtained at the earliest possible moment.

Chronic Dyspepsia, Chronic Gastritis (*Drunkard's Dyspepsia*).—Chronic dyspepsia is caused by repeated attacks of the acute form of this disease; by the excessive use of alcoholic drinks, tea, coffee, or the free use of ice-water during and between meals; by food improperly prepared; by irregularity in eating, imperfect mastication, or excessive tobacco chewing. It also accompanies certain diseases and fevers.

SYMPTOMS.—The principal symptoms of chronic dyspepsia are loss of appetite, constipation, a disagreeable feeling of gnawing and at times a feeling of fullness of the stomach; also tenderness in the stomach, which is but slightly influenced by eating. The stomach becomes prominent from distention, there is occasional nausea and vomiting of a colorless fluid. The tongue is coated, persistent thirst is present, and the patient feels a burning in the pit of the stomach (heartburn) or has pain in the stomach after eating.

When chronic dyspepsia has continued for a considerable time the individual suffers from melancholy and depression of spirits. There may be fainting spells and inability to sleep. Naturally under such conditions there is a loss of weight. With proper treatment most of the symptoms may be greatly relieved, and in many cases a complete cure may be effected.

TREATMENT.—The most essential thing is to correct the diet and by allowing only the proper foods. Avoid fatty, saccharine and starchy articles of diet, discard foods highly seasoned, and use no stimulants of any description.

Milk is beneficial, as are eggs, oysters and a few fresh green vegetables. If a small amount of beef is allowed, give the so-called "Salisbury" steaks. These steaks are made of lean beef, chopped fine, shaped into flattened cakes and broiled. About half-an-hour before eating, the patient should sip slowly a half pint of hot water. This should be repeated before retiring.

For the constipation, any good laxative mineral water is to be recommended.

The hygiene of the body is an important factor in treating chronic dyspepsia. There should be both mental and physical rest, gentle exercise and a change of surroundings.

However, this is a disease that may have serious underlying conditions, and to obtain a positive diagnosis and proper medical treatment the patient should consult a doctor.

Gastric Ulcer, Ulcer of the Stomach.—Ulcer of the stomach occurs most often during early adult life and in females.

SYMPTOMS.—The patient suffers from indigestion, with pain and tenderness in the stomach, vomiting, bleeding from the stomach and extreme acidity of the stomach. The pain comes and goes, and is made worse by taking food, especially if very hot or cold, indigestible or spicy. While the pain is usually located in the pit of the stomach, it may radiate to the back and limbs. Between the pains, dyspepsia is usually present.

Vomiting of undigested food and mucus is common. This may either come directly after eating or about an hour after, according to the location of the ulcer.

If blood is vomited, it is usually dark red, although it may be bright red in color, and in many cases dark-colored blood is passed from the bowels. Anemia, loss of weight and appetite and general failing health accompany the condition.

Ulcer of the stomach develops slowly and runs a regular course, the average duration being about one year. In exceptional cases it develops suddenly. It may end in perforation, peritonitis, fatal hemorrhage or recovery, with the formation of scars. With proper treatment, recoveries are frequent. Relapses are not uncommon.

TREATMENT.—The patient should go to bed and the diet should be only bland foods, such as an ounce or two of milk every two hours with lime water, beef juice, or white of eggs. When feeding by mouth causes too much irritation, the feeding should be by the rectum. (See chapter on Home

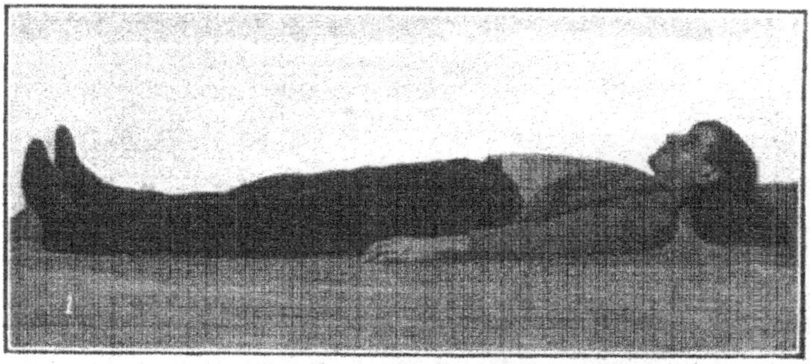

1. POSITION OF PATIENT WHEN THE HEAD SHOULD BE RAISED

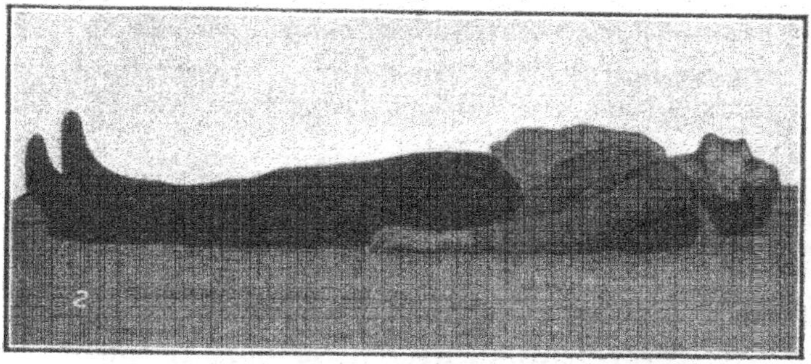

2. POSITION OF PATIENT WHEN HEAD SHOULD BE LOWERED

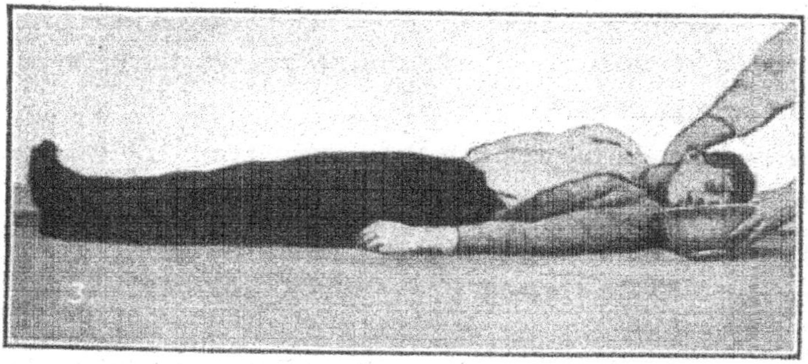

3. POSITION WHEN PATIENT IS VOMITING. THE HEAD IS HELD WELL TO THE SIDE

Nursing.) A nutrient enema should be composed of four ounces of milk, two eggs, a little salt, three drops of the tincture of opium, the entire mixture to be predigested by pancreatin, bought at the drug-store.

If bleeding from the stomach occurs, stop all feeding by mouth and put ice-bags over stomach; pellets of ice internally may be of value.

Hyperacidity is corrected by large doses (about half-a-teaspoonful at a time) of bicarbonate of soda or calcined magnesia, taken every four hours.

For constipation, give some mineral water.

In all cases call a doctor as soon as possible.

Gastric Cancer, Cancer of the Stomach.—Cancer of the stomach, in nearly every case, develops only after forty years of life. It is more frequent in women than in men.

Prolonged irritation, such as accompanies the scars of old ulcers and chronic gastritis, may be predisposing causes.

SYMPTOMS.—Indigestion is present from the beginning. In most cases there is vomiting after eating, and if the stomach becomes dilated from any cause, vomiting will occur. There is frequently bleeding, which is usually only an oozing of dark brown or black blood. This causes a vomit which is characteristic of cancer of the stomach, known as the "coffee grounds" vomit. The oozing blood passes into the intestinal canal and causes bloody stools.

The pain is constant, radiates to the back, is dull and heavy and made worse by the pressure of food,

The patient becomes anemic, there is great emaciation and the rapid loss of weight.

TREATMENT.—Surgical treatment has been of value in some cases; but, as a rule, the only thing to do is to make the patient comfortable. Avoid stimulants, use predigested foods, and, if necessary, resort to feeding by the rectum. (See chapter on Home Nursing.) Cancer of the stomach demands the best medical treatment from the first.

Gastric Dilatation, Dilatation of the Stomach.—Gastric dilatation is an abnormal increase in the cavity of the stomach. Medical advice is indispensable.

SYMPTOMS.—The most characteristic feature of dilatation of the stomach is the vomiting which occurs long after the meals, and often after intervals of several days. The vomit is large in amount and consists of undigested and fermented food and a turbid fluid. In addition to the vomit there may be signs of chronic dyspepsia.

Constipation is common.

Recovery is improbable, but considerable symptomatic relief may be afforded.

TREATMENT.—The diet is important. It should be a "dry" diet, given in small amounts at a time. Fluids should be given by rectal enemas. (See chapter on Home Nursing.) Washing out the stomach every night before bedtime is beneficial. In certain cases surgery can relieve the condition.

Gastric Hemorrhage (*Bleeding from the Stomach*).—

SYMPTOMS.—The principal symptom of this condition is the vomiting of blood.

If the bleeding is from an ulcer of the stomach the blood will be of a bright red color; if from cancer, it will be dark, of the characteristic "coffee grounds" color. (See Ulcer and Cancer of the Stomach.)

If the bleeding is profuse, blood will be noticed in the stools.

The loss of blood will be followed by pallor, weakness, ringing in the ears, faintness and a sinking feeling at the pit of the stomach.

Bleeding from the stomach rarely causes death. In certain diseases it is a grave sign and demands immediate attention from a physican.

TREATMENT.—Put the patient to bed and omit all feeding temporarily. Give ice pellets to swallow and apply ice-bags over stomach and along the spine. In some cases, hot water is equally beneficial. A physician will give medication internally which will allay the condition.

Gastralgia (*Spasm or Neuralgia of the Stomach*).—This is a painful condition of the stomach induced by various forms of irritation, and characterized by violent paroxysms of pain in the stomach.

SYMPTOMS.—There is a severe griping pain in the stomach, usually extending to the back, with a feeling of fainting, a shrunken countenance, and cold hands and feet. The pain becomes so excessive that the patient cries out. The stomach is either puffed out or retracted. External pressure is grateful, and the patient compresses the stomach with his hand.

The attack lasts from a few minutes to half an hour or longer; then the pain gradually subsides, leaving the patient much exhausted, or else it ceases suddenly, with eructation of gas or watery fluid cr with vomiting, and with a gentle, soft perspiration, or with the passage of reddish urine. (Extracts from Romberg's description of an attack.)

TREATMENT.—Apply a hot-water bag over the stomach. Get a doctor immediately. Rest, regulated diet, moderate exercise, fresh air, nerve tonics, etc., are beneficial.

Atonic Dyspepsia ***(Indigestion, Heartburn).***— This very common condition of the American people, especially those who reside in cities, is caused by nervous depression from worry and fatigue, sedentary habits, imperfect mastication, overeating, unchanged diet, heredity, neurasthenia, hysteria, and is found particularly in the female sex.

SYMPTOMS: The appetite is capricious, perverted or lost. Digestion is difficult, and there is a sense of distention and weight in the stomach.

In addition to these signs there may be heartburn, flatulency, regurgitation of portions of partly digested food or acid fluids, water-brash, and pain and soreness in pit of stomach during digestion.

The patient becomes drowsy after meals and suffers from insomnia at night. The memory is defective. There may be headache, lack of mental vigor, flashes of heat, followed by more or less perspiration, and palpitation of the heart. The tongue is usually broad, flabby, pale, and shows the marks of the teeth. The bowels are usually constipated.

1. Nervous Dyspepsia, seen in active business

and professional men, who are nervous and who eat too fast.

2. Flatulent Dyspepsia.—Seen in hysterical individuals.

3. Acid Dyspepsia (*Water Brash*).—Seen when the diet is coarse

4. Irritative Dyspepsia.—Vomiting is a prominent symptom. In these cases the tongue is small, red and pointed.

With proper treatment the outcome is favorable; otherwise the duration is indefinite.

TREATMENT.—The entire living must be changed. In nervous dyspepsia there should be general physical and mental rest. The diet should be regulated and should contain in the foods little or no sugars, starch or fats.

Special attention should be paid to mastication, which must be slow and complete and only small quantities of food taken at a time.

Under-done meat, "Salisbury steaks," eggs, fish, oysters, green vegetables and stale or brown bread are advised.

No stimulants should be taken with the meals and only small quantities of fluids.

To rest for half an hour after meals is a good plan.

For cases of dyspepsia, where acidity of the

stomach is obvious, a simple and efficacious remedy is bicarbonate of soda, taken either in its dry condition or dissolved in water.

DISEASES OF THE INTESTINES

Intestinal Indigestion.—Intestinal indigestion may be inherited or due to a bad diet, over-eating or irregularity in time of eating, deficient exercise, worry and a tired-out brain; excessive use of tobacco or stimulants, or diseases of the stomach, liver or pancreas, or malaria may induce intestinal indigestion.

Symptoms.—There are two forms of intestinal indigestion—acute and chronic.

Acute Form.—In this variety there is severe loss of appetite, headache and diarrhœa.

When the attack is sudden, the gases that accumulate cause attacks of colic. In these cases there is a feeling of weariness, with chills, fever, coated tongue, pains in the abdomen increased by pressure, cramps in the legs, diarrhœa and headache with or without vomiting.

Chronic Form.—In this variety the pain does not come on until from two to six hours after eating, with tenderness and distention in the upper part of the abdomen. There is also shortness of the breath with constipation. As the affection progresses, the patient becomes anemic, loses weight and grows nervous.

TREATMENT: *Acute Form.*—Give two grains of calomel in doses of a quarter of a grain every fifteen minutes and follow six hours after the last dose with salts.

Chronic Form.—In this form some good laxative water should be used daily.

The diet should be regulated. It should be small in amount and confined to articles easily digested in the stomach, as beef, eggs and milk.

Intestinal Colic (*Gripes*).—Colic of the intestines may be due to constipation, the presence of indigestible food, an abnormal quantity of bile in the intestinal tract, or to certain diseases.

SYMPTOMS.—Severe pain of a tearing, ripping, twisting, pinching or bearing-down character, centering about the umbilicus (the navel) is the most prominent symptom. The abdomen becomes tense and pressure will relieve the pain.

When the attack is very severe, the body-surface is bathed in a cold sweat, the features are pinched and nausea and vomiting may add to the discomfort of the patient. Constipation is usually present. The duration of an attack of intestinal colic is from a few minutes to several hours. A discharge of gas is the usual termination.

Treatment.—During attack give a half grain of calomel every half hour until four grains are taken. Follow in six hours with a dose of salts.

Constipation.—Constipation may be due to many causes, among which may be mentioned diseases of the digestive tract, fevers, affections that diminish the wave-like movement of the intestines, sedentary habits, neglecting to move the bowels at regular intervals, improper food, malaria, lead-poisoning, displaced organs, or foreign bodies.

Symptoms.—Constipation in one person would not be called such in another. It is a relative term. A person used to two stools a day, might become constipated should he suddenly change to one stool. One stool in twenty-four hours is normal for the vast majority of people, and constipation is likely to result when stools are less frequent than this.

When a person is truly constipated there will be straining, distress and irritation of the rectum. These signs are shortly followed by symptoms of dyspepsia, such as headache, fainting, palpitation of the heart and often abdominal distention.

Treatment.—Have the cause of the constipation discovered and removed. Success in treating constipation rests largely with the patient.

If the following suggestions are adopted, constipation may be greatly relieved:

Have regular hours for evacuating the bowels and stay long enough for them to be emptied. If necessary, assist nature with a warm water injection until daily stools become a habit, but beware of becoming dependent upon any artificial helps in this matter.

Regulate the diet carefully and confine it mainly to vegetables, fruits, brown bread, gluten bread, plenty of water, corn meal and oat meal, until relief is obtained and regular evacuations are established.

A daily dose of purgative mineral waters is recommended. Epsom or Rochelle salts are equally good.

Daily bathing and exercise will do much to restore a normal condition.

Electricity and kneading of the abdominal walls or massage will restore the tone of the abdominal muscles. Persistent constipation may be due to intestinal obstruction, a very grave condition; therefore, if the bowels do not move for three or four days, the safest plan is to consult a physician.

Diarrhœa.—Diarrhœa may be caused by indigestion, by indigestible or impure food or water, by irritating matters or secretions poured into the bowels or by intestinal inflammation. Atmospheric changes, sudden mental shock, purgatives, certain infectious fevers and other diseases also cause diarrhœa.

SYMPTOMS.—Diarrhœa may be either acute or may run a chronic course.

Acute Form.—The patient, a few hours after eating, experiences colicky pains in the abdomen; he is nauseated, his tongue is coated and he has a desire for stool. Purging relieves the pain. The stools are very offensive. Their color becomes lighter after four or five evacuations. The duration of the attack is usually from two to four days.

There is a variety of diarrhœa, in which the food passes through unaltered or very slightly digested. The stools are frequent and emaciation is common.

In another variety griping pains are felt in the abdomen, scalding sensations at the anus, and the stools are green or yellow.

Chronic Form.—Chronic diarrhœa results from the persistence of the acute form or from constitutional affections.

The stools continue to be frequent, but are paler in color. Accompanying this form, emaciation, anemia and dyspepsia occur.

A diarrhœa is nothing but a symptom and its cessation depends upon the underlying conditions.

TREATMENT.—In the acute form, cease work as nature suggests. Administer a laxative, as castor oil or salts. Restrict the diet to pure boiled milk and lime water for a few days. Then resume the usual diet gradually.

If the affection persists or threatens to become chronic, a doctor's skill is needed to treat the condition.

Intestinal Catarrh (*Inflammation of the Bowels*).—There are many causes of inflammation of the bowels. A few of the most frequent causes are contagious or poisonous matter, ptomaine poisoning, exposure to cold or wet while perspiring, irritants, such as foreign bodies in the intestinal tract, and imperfect hygiene.

SYMPTOMS: *Acute Form.*—The affection begins with a feeling of lassitude. The patient has chills, loss of appetite, fever, colicky pains, localized abdominal tenderness, nausea and vomiting.

At first the bowels are constipated; later there is a diarrhœa. The stools may become very frequent, thin and watery—the so-called "rice water" discharge.

Chronic Form.—In addition to the diarrhœa,

emaciation and anemia supervene. The stools are thin, watery and frequent.

The outcome is favorable when the treatment is prompt and appropriate. Mild cases last four or five days; severe cases from one to two weeks.

In the chronic form, diarrhœa may persist indefinitely.

TREATMENT.—Put the patient to bed and restrict the diet to milk with lime water and mutton or chicken broths with well-boiled rice.

At the beginning, give two grains of calomel in doses of a quarter of a grain every fifteen minutes and follow six hours after last dose with citrate of magnesia or Epsom salts. If the symptoms become severe it is necessary to have medical aid at once.

In chronic cases attention should be given to the clothing and hygiene. Locally, poultices or camphorated oil are beneficial.

Cholera Morbus (*Bilious Cholera, English Cholera*).—Cholera morbus is most frequent in the summer and early autumn, although in the tropics the disease is likely to occur at any time. It may be caused by sudden changes in the temperature, the eating of unripe fruit or vegetables, and the presence of irritants in the digestive tract.

SYMPTOMS: The onset of this disease is sudden and violent, occurring, as a rule, after midnight.

The patient experiences a chilly sensation, intense nausea, vomiting and purging, accompanied by distressing burning or tearing abdominal pains or colic.

At first, the vomit consists of ordinary stomach contents, but afterward of bilious material, and later of almost pure water.

The stools are frequent; at first ordinary in character, then of whitish or greenish liquid and later "rice-water."

The surface of the body is cold and covered with a clammy sweat. In severe cases, intense muscular cramps are present. The patient becomes rapidly weak and emaciated, and collapse may occur.

As a rule, the outlook is favorable, the attack lasting in mild cases only one or two days. In severe cases, it may last one or more weeks, followed by a tedious convalescence. During infancy and old age, the outcome is likely to be fatal.

TREATMENT.—Put the patient to bed, cease all feeding and call a doctor.

Acute Dysentery (*Bloody Flux*).—Acute Dysentery may be caused by changes in climate, errors in diet, impure drinking water, exposure to wet and cold and bad hygiene. It occurs most often during the summer and autumn seasons.

SYMPTOMS.—The affection begins gradually. At first there is a diarrhœa, the patient loses his appetite, is nauseated and has a slight fever, which continues for two or three days, when the true symptoms develop. These symptoms are pain on pressure along the upper part and down the left side of the abdomen, or colicky pains about the navel and burning pains in the rectum, with the feeling of the presence of a foreign body, and a constant desire to expel it.

For the first two days the stools are normal in consistency, but very soon change to a grayish, tough, transparent mucus, containing more or less blood and pus. In number, they vary from five to twenty in twenty-four hours.

In another form the stools are not so many, but the emaciation is marked.

There is a croupous variety of acute dysentery, which has a rapid onset. The stools are frequent, with nausea and vomiting, great prostration and emaciation. The skin is cold and the patient emits a disagreeable odor. Gaseous distention of the abdomen is common and the fever is high.

Chronic Dysentery.—In the chronic variety there is a persistence in the intestinal lesions of any of the acute forms. Diarrhœa and emaciation are the principal symptoms. The abdominal pain is slight. The attack may last several months or even years.

TREATMENT.—Even in the mildest attacks, put the patient to bed and employ the bed-pan. After using the bed-pan, thoroughly disinfect it

Give the patient a bland, unirritating diet, composed of milk, with lime water, beef peptonoids, broths, egg albumens, etc., in acute cases.

In chronic cases use a semi-solid diet. In all cases of dysentery known or suspected, a doctor should be called without delay.

Proctitis (*Catarrh of the Rectum*).—This condition results from constipation, from the habitual use of enemas and purgatives, from diseases of the liver, piles or sitting on damp ground or stone steps.

SYMPTOMS.—There is a burning pain in the rectum with a desire to evacuate, and hardened feces or stools containing mucus, muco-pus or blood are passed.

There may also be present nausea, headache, fever and a heavy, tired feeling.

In simple cases the outlook is favorable.

TREATMENT.—The constipation should be relieved by a soap-suds enema (see chapter on Home

Nursing) or an enema composed of the following:

Magnesium sulphate.......2 ounces
Glycerin.............one-half ounce
Boiled water ....4 ounces

Hot injections of strong black coffee, using from half a pint to a quart, are valuable when the rectum is irritable and there is a tendency to diarrhœa.

Occasionally, cold injections are more beneficial.

Intestinal Obstruction or Occlusion.—Intestinal obstruction is a sudden or gradual closure of the intestinal canal, characterized by pain, nausea, vomiting, constipation and finally collapse.

SYMPTOMS.—The acute symptoms of intestinal obstruction are spasmodic abdominal pain, becoming continuous in character.

Constipation which is unrelieved by purgatives or enemas. The abdomen becomes greatly distended and very tender in spots; there is nausea and a characteristic vomit.

As the condition progresses, the features become pinched, the eyes sunken, the skin cold and clammy and there are present other signs of collapse.

Chronic cases have as signs obstinate constipation, with the passage of ribbon-shaped stools, abdominal pain and failure in health. The onset is gradual, and a chronic case may become acute when the obstruction is complete.

The possible outcome is so grave that the services of a physician must be procured immediately, who will prescribe treatment.

Treatment.—Give no drugs by mouth to move the bowels. Withhold all foods.

If necessary give nutrient enemas to sustain the patient. (See chapter on Home Nursing.)

Tape-Worms.—Tape-worms are caused by eating meats and fish infected by the tape-worm, which are improperly cooked and prepared.

Symptoms.—Very often there are no symptoms. As a rule, the patient has colicky pains, a ferocious appetite, trouble with digestion, he loses weight, becomes anemic and constipated, and in some cases has fainting spells and itching of the arms and nose. When he eats a large meal, the symptoms cease.

The presence of a piece of tape-worm in the stools confirms the diagnosis.

Treatment.—Restrict the diet to liquids for two days. Give the patient two grains of calomel, in doses of a quarter of a grain every fifteen minutes, and follow it six hours later with a dose of salts. Then give half a teaspoonful of the oleoresin of aspidium (never give any oil following aspidium), and after it acts give another two grains of calomel. Watch the stools for the head of the tape-worm.

The best plan to follow, if the presence of a tape-worm is suspected, is to call a physician.

Round Worms.—There are several varieties of round worms, each one giving a different set of symptoms, and each one requiring special treatment.

SYMPTOMS.—A positive diagnosis can be made only upon the passage of the parasite.

Some of the leading symptoms are: Picking of the nose, foul breath, colicky pains, disturbed sleep, grinding the teeth and itching about the anus.

Should the parasites migrate to the sexual organs, intense itching is caused, and unless discovered in time and corrected, bad habits may follow in the case of children.

TREATMENT.—See a competent physician and follow his treatment. Ignorant experiments with this affection are dangerous.

Biliousness (*Torpid Liver*).—Biliousness may be caused by atmospheric or artificial heat, chronic constipation, excessive use of alcohol, or malaria. In females an arrested menstrual period may give rise to an attack.

SYMPTOMS.—This affection begins with a feeling

of lassitude and depression of spirits, accompanied by pains in the legs, headache, a coated tongue, loss of appetite, nausea, and very often vomiting. Constipation and flatulence are present, and the complexion is muddy. As a rule, the attack lasts about a week.

TREATMENT.—If the attack is caused by errors of diet the following mixture should be given:

Bicarbonate of soda....... 5 grains
Powdered ipecac .....one-half grain
Calomel ....3 grains

Take at one dose and follow in two hours with half an ounce of magnesium sulphate or a teaspoonful of sodium phosphate in half a glass of water.

Hot applications over the region of the liver may be tried.

For several days restrict the diet to liquids and soft foods, such as toast, chicken, eggs and breakfast foods.

CHAPTER VII

DISEASES OF THE NERVOUS SYSTEM

Most nervous diseases are too obscure and complicated to be treated in a book of this character. As, however, neurotic individuals, children as well as adults, are increasing in number as our civilization and mode of life become more complex, it is necessary to say something of the symptoms which give warning of impending nervous diseases.

Headache.—Headaches are divided into classes as to their occurrence: persistent, periodically recurrent, and occasional. A persistent, long continued headache is usually due to some organic disease. This disease may be in the brain itself, as a tumor or brain abscess, or in some other part of the body. In middle-aged people, a constant headache sometimes indicates Bright's disease of the kidneys. The important point is that when a person has a persistent headache he may be sure he has a serious sickness and should consult a doctor as soon as possible.

Periodically recurring headache is usually due

to some functional disorder. In other words, the machinery of the body is not running smoothly. The most usual forms of this are Migraine or Sick Headache and Neuralgia. There are other less frequent forms called Tic Douloureux and Brow Ague.

Migraine is usually on one side of the head only. It is preceded by a series of sensations which warn the sufferer that he is to have one of these attacks. Sometimes there is partial blindness or dizziness or simply a feeling that the head is very full and throbbing. After an hour or two the headache begins. This is one-sided, usually concentrating on the eyes and brow. The pain is intense, the patient is prostrated, faint and nauseated. Any food which has been eaten recently is vomited undigested, and this vomiting continues until bile is thrown out. At this point, the patient begins to feel better, generally falls asleep and awakes well. During the attack the flow of saliva is increased, and a large quantity of pale urine is passed. The entire attack takes from six to eight hours. There is no set time for these headaches to recur, but they usually follow some form of exhaustion of the nerve centres. Severe study, loss of sleep, sudden anxiety or great social excitement tend to bring on the attacks. Some people seem to have recurrences at times of disturbed digestion or at the menstrual period. They are more common in women than in men. These attacks begin in childhood or youth, and in spite of treatment continue, gradually diminishing in frequency and force as middle age is reached.

These headaches may be an inherited weakness, but changing from an indoor city life to an outdoor country existence, is frequently enough to stop or at least markedly diminish these attacks. When the attacks begin, the possibility of an inflamed appendix or gall-bladder should be considered, and a doctor should be called. But after a person has had a few of these headaches he can generally treat himself better than any one else. He knows to what relief his particular migraine yields the quickest.

It is necessary to warn the reader against the numerous headache remedies now on the market. They are powerful depressants of the heart and have been known to cause serious injury. Let some good doctor prescribe instead. During the attack take no food or drink, as either will probably be vomited and will only serve to increase the irritation. An exception may be made in favor of hot strong tea or coffee, without milk or sugar. These sometimes give relief, or at least mitigate pain. These headaches are sometimes due to eye trouble; an oculist should be consulted.

Neuralgia.—Neuralgia is a recurring attack of pain in some of the nerves of the head, usually the fifth nerve. The attacks are usually on one side and recur at the same time of the day. The pain is sharp, darting and very severe, and there are often tender spots along the course of the nerve. The cause of this painful malady is not always clear, but many general conditions predispose to it. Thus, an anemic person will often suffer from neuralgia until the blood condition has been corrected. Eye-strain unnoticed and uncorrected is also a potent factor, as are diseased teeth. In women who suffer from chronic constipation and leucorrhœa neuralgia often appears. Gouty or rheumatic irritation of the nerves will predispose to neuralgia. In treating any neuralgia, all these things must be considered and the general cause sought for and treated. The pain of an attack is often so severe that drugs have to be given to relieve the sufferer. These should be taken on a doctor's prescription, as they are powerful, and dangerous unless used properly. In the general treatment an iron tonic, good purgatives and fresh air and sunshine, not forgetting good, wholesome food, go a long way toward curing most people.

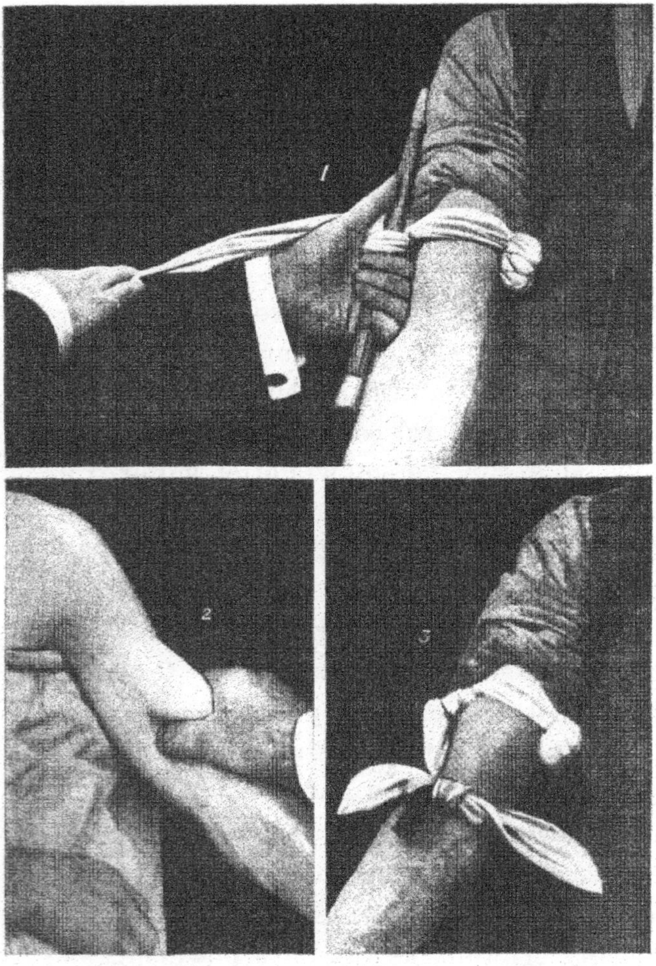

1. APPLYING A TOURNIQUET TO THE UPPER ARM TO CONTROL BLEEDING AT A LOWER POINT

2. PRESSURE BY THUMB OF THE MAIN ARTERY OF THE ARM TO CONTROL BLEEDING

3. THE TOURNIQUET FINISHED AND IN PLACE

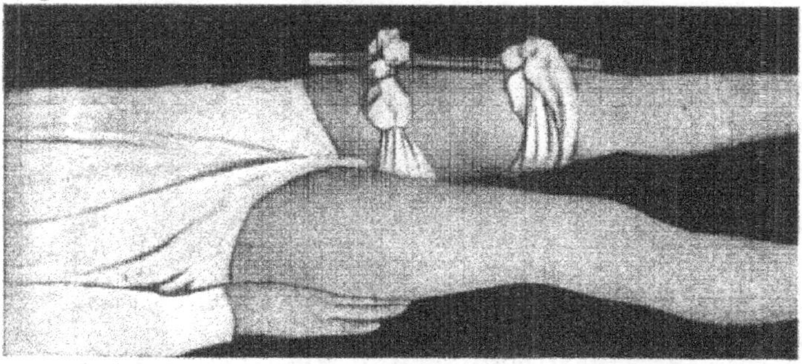

1. TOURNIQUET OF THIGH TO CONTROL BLEEDING BELOW THAT POINT

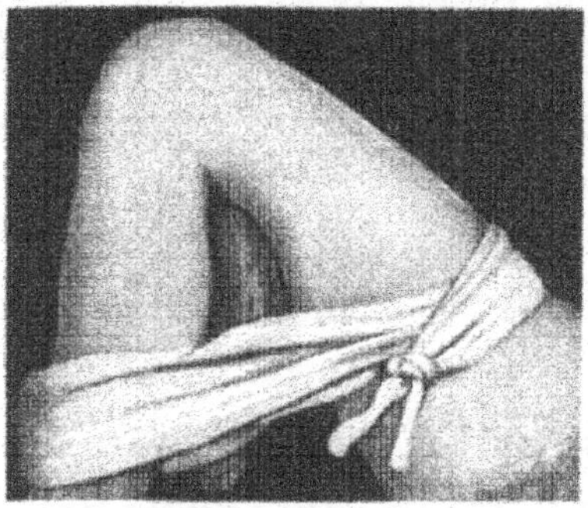

2. PADDING BEHIND KNEE AND ACUTE FLEXION OF KNEE TO CONTROL BLEEDING BEHIND KNEE

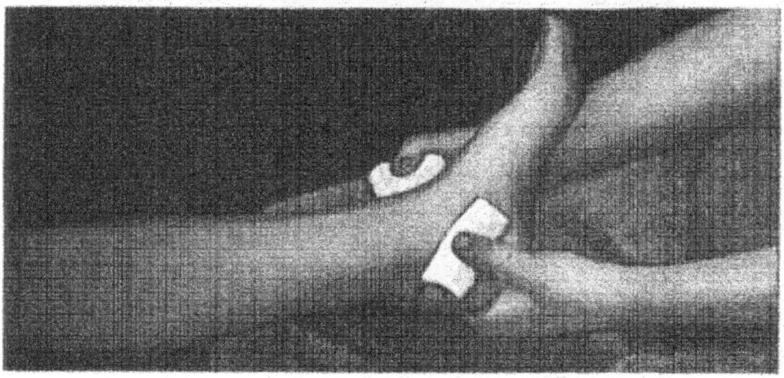

3. PRESSURE APPLIED OVER ARTERY TO THE FOOT TO CONTROL BLEEDING

It is unnecessary to go into detail about the rarer forms of recurring head pains. In most cases, rest and quiet with some simple sedative are the best remedies. A drug habit is very easily formed in such cases, so it is well to be very careful in the administering of drugs.

Brow Ague occurs in people who have had malaria for a long time. It affects the nerve, which runs up the forehead from the orbit. It is periodical in time and very severe in character. It is treated best by quinine, arsenic and iron, prescribed in all cases by a physician.

Tic Douloureux is an acute form of neuralgia, which affects the fifth nerve usually, although it may attack others. The pain lasts only a moment or so, but may appear at very short intervals. The cause of this neuralgia is obscure. The patient's condition is pitiable. He can do nothing; the suffering is so intense, that often people have been driven to suicide. The disease is, fortunately, rare.

Occasional Headaches are due to a great variety of causes, usually functional. They appear irregularly and are not localized or of a specific character. The presence of toxins in the blood, resulting from bad food or more often constipation, is a potent source of this kind of headache.

The continued breathing of bad air will bring on a severe headache. In some women at the menstrual period there is a sharp headache, supposed to be due to a toxic condition. A headache with fever is common. This is best treated by cold sponging and an ice-cap.

A Fatigue Headache is a common experience. The treatment of this is obvious. Rest is the sovereign remedy. A cup of coffee acts as a stimulant at such times and is very beneficial.

The student gets a dull headache frequently, combined with cold hands and feet. He needs fresh air and exercise to correct his way of living.

In general, this form of headache needs and should get no drug. The danger of forming a habit is too great.

Insomnia.—Insomnia means involuntary wakefulness. There are various forms of it and various causes. Most people have experienced an occasional insomnia, lasting one or two nights, or at least a partial insomnia, in which hours of wakefulness are succeeded at last by sleep. Some physiological error is usually the cause of this. The person suffering from insomnia of this kind may be over-fatiguing himself or he may have been eating indigestible food late at night. On the other hand, if he has not eaten for five or six hours it may be his empty stomach which is keeping him awake. Excessive use of tobacco, tea or coffee also tend to insomnia. The only treatment of this form is to correct the bad habit which is causing it.

Any unusual circumstance about the surroundings is enough to produce insomnia in some people. Undue heat, cold, noise or light, or an unusual position maintained constantly will cause a wakeful night.

Insomnia is a very trying symptom of some diseases in their early form. Pneumonia, typhoid, pleurisy and some forms of heart disease all have insomnia in their beginnings, and in cases such as these the doctor in charge will always give an opiate. A good night's rest is more valuable in that stage of the disease than any other treatment.

Insomnia occurs in cases of anemia and in some other constitutional illnesses; also it sometimes precedes acute attacks of insanity. Sometimes the effect on the patient is so great that drugs must be resorted to, but this should *never* be done without a doctor's advice, and the person who is to take the drug should never know what it is. It is from this class of people that a large percentage of "drug fiends" come. There is nothing so pitiable as a person who cannot sleep. Such a one, when once he learns of a drug which will help him, is powerless to resist taking it.

Unless an attack is of a passing character consult a physician promptly. The condition is one requiring trained judgment and care.

Sea-Sickness, Mal-de-Mer.—Any one who has ever experienced it knows what sea-sickness means. Some people suffer only slightly; others may be seriously ill. Some may recover after a few days and experience no return; others will continue to suffer and never seem to grow accustomed to the sea.

SYMPTOMS.—The symptoms are always headache, nausea and vomiting, and a feeling of depression which may amount to collapse. The cause seems to be in the unaccustomed and continued motion, with all the shaking up of the internal organs which that implies, and the confused visual sensation accompanying such motion. Many people experience the same feeling in train-traveling, and also temporary sensations of a similar kind in a swing, a hammock and when descending or ascending in an elevator.

The sea-sick victim becomes white and clammy cold; he vomits and has the most intense feeling of continued nausea. Diarrhœa often accompanies this vomiting. Severe headache and complete nervous collapse are common. Most people, in the course of time, outgrow these symptoms and become perfectly well.

TREATMENT.—Any one who knows he is easily affected should take precautions before beginning any sea trip. Good general health is the first and best preventive. Have the bowels open and the stomach in good shape. Before going on board, a full dose of bromide is often helpful. Have your doctor give it to you. Then when you reach the boat lie down as near the centre of the ship as is possible, with the head low and toward the bow. A full meal should have been eaten before going on board. And, in general, do not let your stomach get empty, as that is conducive to sea-sickness. Good sized doses (30 to 60 drops) of aromatic spirits of ammonia are successful with many people. Unless the attack is very severe and the patient does not recover promptly no medical assistance is needed.

Nervousness.—Many people, especially women, find as they grow older that they are "nervous." By this they mean that little things upset them easily; they are over-emotional, laughing or crying at trivial matters; they cannot enjoy life; They are irritated and "on edge" over everything. These people seek a doctor for relief.

What has brought about this condition? Almost always a prolonged period of great physical and mental strain or some sudden shock. Nursing a chronic case of illness is one of the very usual means by which a woman becomes exhausted nervously. The constant care, attention and the willing sacrifice of strength, sleep and fresh air, all assist in the breakdown. The busy mother who for years has worried along, raising a large family on too little money, with all the planning and worrying that entails, is another person who is likely to suffer from a severe nervous collapse, or at least a general nervousness, which unfits her for many of the duties she hitherto exercised.

The suddenness of a great loss or of a terrifying physical experience has often unstrung the healthiest of beings for months (men as well as women). But it is well understood that women suffer mostly from these conditions.

What is to be done about these matters? A little knowledge and a good deal of common sense would save many a long doctor's bill, many a month lost in ill health and suffering.

If a person is to be under some such prolonged strain, let some one in the family see to it that that person lives correctly. Insist on a certain number of hours of undisturbed sleep, a certain amount of fresh air and mild exercise and proper eating, bathing, etc. Under these conditions, a person stands the strain and the hard physical work much better and longer, and feels less nervous exhaustion in the end.

When it is seen that the prolonged strain is beginning to tell too severely, be warned in time. Insist that the person cease from her exertions entirely, if possible. But, if not, at least mitigate them. Remember, that a woman who makes herself a chronic invalid for life, for the sake of a few months of effort, is not really helping her family. Here is where common sense comes in.

Any shocking news or word of some loss should be broken gently whenever possible. Most people understand that this should be done, even if they do not fully understand the psychological reasons for it.

Dr. S. Weir Mitchell speaks of such a thing as a moral wound which must heal just as a bodily wound must heal.

In bringing up their children, especially girls, wise mothers will note early the evidences of nervousness and will make every effort to overcome them. Bring up your girls to live healthy out-of-door lives and do not crowd them too fast in their studies. At the sensitive period of puberty, when the girl changes from a child to a young woman, special care must be taken of her.

Early in life the standards of conduct for boys and girls are taught differently. The boy is taught self-control, physical courage, truthfulness. The girl is taught modesty and good manners. Each child should be taught more of what the other gets. Girls need the training in self-control and physical courage. Boys need the training in personal modesty and the gentler habits of life. Boys and girls will be better men and women when they are trained more nearly along the same correct lines of conduct.

Insanity.—Little need be said here of this dreadful disease, which has wrecked so many homes. Some forms of insanity are so apparent that any one can make the diagnosis, but there are other types in which the patient is so sane on all subjects at certain times as to defy detection, except by a trained observer of the insane. Where there is any suspicion of insanity it is only just, not only to the community and family, but to the patient himself, to call in medical aid immediately. Prompt and correct treatment has cured many cases.

A great mistake is often made in keeping the afflicted person at home and attempting to care for him by members of the family. This is, of course, because people feel that there is some disgrace in having insanity in the family and the fear that the loved relative may not be treated kindly enough in an institution. This viewpoint is wrong. Insanity is a disease not so well understood as some others, but still responding to the same general line of treatment. The home atmosphere, full of loving indulgence and misguided kindness, is often the very worst place for the sufferer. He or she needs the impersonal, routine life of a sanitarium or asylum, with the care of people trained to understand the diseased mind. Then, too, we must remember that this home care often means the sacrifice of the health of the one member of the family on whom the care of the patient falls heaviest. Nothing is so sad as the sight of these devoted but misguided relatives giving their very lives to a hopeless cause. It is the part of wisdom and common sense to take the advice of the trained outsider, the family doctor or specialist, and let him guide the patient's course of treatment.

Epilepsy.—Epilepsy is supposed to be a disease of the brain. It is usually inherited either from epileptic parents or those who have been drunkards, insane, hysterical, etc., and it develops during the formative period of the brain.

Symptoms.—Epilepsy is characterized by sudden loss of consciousness, accompanied by more or less general convulsions. It is divided into the "*grand mal*" and the "*petit mal*," (big and little sickness). In *grand mal* there is a sudden premonition of the coming attack, called the aura, and then the patient falls, with a peculiar cry, and becomes unconscious. The face is pale and the body rigid. This is followed by convulsions for a while. Then the patient becomes quiet and lies in a deep stupor. Often he bites his tongue in an attack, or otherwise injures himself in falling.

In the *petit mal* the patient may have a feeling of dizziness or a period of confused absent-mindedness, lasting for a minute or two.

Treatment.—Any epileptic should be under a doctor's care, for it is only by care and efficient treatment that there is any chance for a cure.

However, every one should know what to do when a patient is suddenly attacked and a physician is not available.

First of all, insert something in the mouth to prevent the tongue from being bitten. A spoon wrapped in a handkerchief, a towel wadded into a thick piece or a clothes-pin will do—anything, in fact, which is too large to be swallowed. Next, remove anything against which the patient may strike and injure himself. If any one can procure an amyl nitrite pearl from a drug-store, break it in a handkerchief and let the patient inhale it. Otherwise wait for the attack to pass off and then let the patient sleep.

CHAPTER VIII

DISEASES OF EYE, EAR, NOSE AND THROAT

THE eye and the ear are such delicate organs that when anything goes wrong, it is unwise for any one not especially trained to try to treat them. Even general practitioners refer most of this work to specialists. But, *always remembering how much harm can be done and how delicate the eye and ear are,* a few of the simplest injuries and ailments may be described and their treatment outlined.

Cinders or Foreign Bodies in the Eye.—Foreign bodies may lodge beneath the lower or upper lids or on the eyeball itself. If beneath the lower lid, there is little or no pain, because the lid is loose and gives easily. But, if beneath the upper lid, where there is greater pressure against the eyeball, the accident is very painful and dangerous, for with every movement of the lid a tiny scratch is made on the eyeball. This may result in an ulcer, if long continued. Similarly, if the cinder is imbedded in the eyeball itself, the pain is intense and the result of its continued pressure there may be an ulcer or an inflammation of the eyeball.

Treatment.—If the cinder has just entered the eye and can be readily seen, it is usually possible to remove it by holding the lids apart, locating the cinder and wiping it out with a quick dab of the edge of a clean handkerchief or with absorbent cotton. If the cinder cannot be seen, it is probably under the upper lid. Have the patient look steadfastly toward the ground. Then take hold of the eyelashes of the upper lid. Place a pencil or any small stick across the upper lid and roll the lid over it, exposing the under surface. When the cinder is discovered remove it with a piece of cotton or clean linen. To allay the irritation caused, it is well to irrigate the eye with boric acid solution.

Sometimes a cinder or minute fragment of steel is imbedded in the eyeball and must be picked out with a needle. Before this can be done, the eye must be made insensitive to pain and touch. Several drops of a 2 per cent. solution of cocaine will do this completely. The needle used should be previously cleaned by lying in 95 per cent. alcohol for at least ten minutes. The picking must be done very carefully, and an unskilled person should never attempt the feat if a doctor can be secured. After the cinder is out, the eye should be washed every hour for a day or so with a few drops of boric acid solution (a teaspoonful to a glass of water).

Ecchymosis (*Black Eye*).—The condition called a "black eye," is simply a bruise of the tissues around the eye. Being very soft, they swell easily and excessively. For the same reason the small arteries and veins easily rupture and there is excessive discoloration.

TREATMENT.—Reduction of the swelling is the first thing to be done. Apply cloths wrung out of ice water to the eye continually, or else lay little round pieces of linen on a piece of ice. When these are ice-cold apply them, changing them as they warm up. After the swelling has gone down, apply very hot applications, which will hasten the removal of the discoloration. Do not apply an oyster or other poultice, as this will do no good and may cause infection.

Wounds and Burns of the Eye.—Slight wounds or burns of the eye or lid will heal readily, if boric acid solution is put in the eyes every few hours for several days. But any injury which is not obviously very slight should receive the attention of a doctor immediately.

Hordeolum (*Stye*).—A stye is a boil on the eyelid. It begins as a hard, painful red swelling of the eyelid. After a time the tip becomes yellow, ruptures and discharges "matter" or pus. If an eyelash can be seen coming out of the top of the swelling, to remove it with forceps will hasten the subsidence of the stye.

TREATMENT.—To bathe the stye every three or four hours with hot boric acid solution will hasten the formation of "matter" and hence the cure of the stye. If one stye follows another, this fact indicates a general condition of poor health. A physician should be seen and a tonic prescribed. Eye-strain will sometimes cause an irritation which may result in styes.

Congestion of the Eyelids.—This condition may be caused by dust or foreign bodies in the eye, by exposure to glaring light, by reading in a poor light constantly, and frequently by eye-strain. A germ infection also will cause a congestion.

The eyes are tired, they smart and "feel as if sand were in them." The lids are slightly swollen and reddened on their inner side.

TREATMENT.—Rest the eyes, use dark glasses, and wash the eyes with boric acid solution. If in a few days they are not cured, see an oculist without delay.

Conjunctivitis, Catarrhal Inflammation of the Eyes (*Sore Eyes*).—This condition sometimes follows a simple congestion and is a more severe form of it. It is almost always due to a germ infection and is contagious.

The lids and conjunctiva (lining of the lids and eyeball) are swollen, red and painful. There is a discharge which makes the lids stick together over night. Sight is not at first interfered with, except that light causes so much pain that the patient will not use his eyes.

In some specific infections of the eye, a thick creamy pus is discharged. This is very dangerous and may result in blindness, unless treated promptly and by a physician. But immediate home treatment may save some patients' eyes. This last form is most commonly seen in babies only a few days old.

"Pink eye" is another contagious form of conjunctivitis. The symptoms and treatment are similar.

Treatment.—Irrigate the eyes frequently with boric acid solution, or even with warm salt solution, a teaspoonful to a pint of water. Keep iced compresses on the eyes constantly. Keep the patient quiet and in a darkened room, so that the eyes are not used at all. When matter comes from the eyes, a drop of 1 per cent. solution of silver nitrate should be put in the eyes twice a day and followed immediately by boric acid or salt solution. The rest of the treatment is as above. But do not fail to get a doctor immediately. Any delay may cause a permanent loss of sight.

If only one eye is involved, the well eye should be carefully protected from infection. It should be covered with a clean cloth and bandaged before treating the sick eye.

Eye-Strain.—This is a general term which includes the effect on the eye of near-sightedness, far-sightedness and astigmatism. No discussion of it is possible in this place, but a short account of its symptoms may be given, so that the intelligent reader may be warned in time when it is wise to seek an oculist.

Headache is a very usual symptom of eye-strain. This may take any form. Dizziness, nausea and vomiting may also occur, especially after the eyes have been used for some time. "Cross eye" which comes and goes, is another symptom showing weakness of the eye muscles.

In consulting a doctor for eye-strain, go to a specialist, for he is most competent to handle these cases.

Deafness, Sudden and Gradual.—Sudden deafness is frequently due to an accumulation of wax in the ears. There is a normal amount of wax in all ears, though some have more than others. If water finds its way into the outer ear and causes the wax to swell the canal will be quickly closed and deafness result. There is usually dizziness, and noises of an annoying kind will be heard in the deaf ear.

The best way to remove the wax is to put a few drops of a strong solution of sodium bicarbonate (baking soda) (two teaspoonfuls to half a glass of water) into the ear and then a small wad of cotton. Leave this for a day and night and the wax will be thoroughly softened. Then take a solution of sodium bicarbonate (a teaspoonful to a pint of water) and with a small syringe of hard or soft rubber irrigate the ear repeatedly until at last the mass of wax comes out. This may take some time, but the irrigation can do no harm if it is not done too forcibly, and it should be kept up until the mass comes away. When finished the ear should be dried with cotton and a piece of cotton worn in the ear for a day or so.

Gradual deafness is generally due to a catarrhal inflammation of the middle ear or of some other structure of the ear. There is no place in a book such as this for any discussion of such a chronic condition. Treatment by an ear specialist is the only thing to be recommended.

Earache.—Earache is usually due to an acute inflammation of the middle ear. This may subside or may go on to an abscess, when the drum of the ear ruptures and pus is discharged, *i. e.*, the ear "runs." This abscess occurs in what is known as the middle ear. The middle ear communicates with the back of the throat by means of the Eustachian tube. Hence, any throat trouble, such as adenoids, enlarged tonsils, chronic catarrhal trouble or severe "colds" of nose and throat are likely to infect the middle ear and cause an abscess.

Douching of the nose or spraying, except with the proper apparatus, is therefore very dangerous, as it may force infection up the Eustachian tubes. Blowing the nose violently during a cold, and sniffing up solutions, are dangerous for the same reason. An unskilful person should not attempt any local treatment until a physician has examined the patient. To alleviate violent pain, the patient should lie with the affected side on a very hot water bag. The external ear may be douched with hot salt solution (a teaspoonful of salt to a pint of water). This is to be done very gently and the ear dried after each douching. Ten drops of laudanum for a grown person, or half a teaspoonful of paregoric for a child, may be given, if the pain is extreme and no doctor can be procured. Do not delay to have a doctor see the patient, for the hearing may be saved, at least in part, if the doctor cuts the ear-drum instead of letting it rupture by itself. Never use patent "ear drops," and never put oily substances in the ear to relieve pain or inflammation.

Foreign Bodies in the Ear.—Children often put buttons, beans, etc., in their ears, and sometimes insects find their way into the external ear. These latter cause intense suffering by their struggles to escape. The irritation of the drum makes the victim hear constant noise and almost drives him out of his mind.

The quickest way to remove an insect is to drop sweet oil, linseed oil or even glycerine in the ear and then douche it out immediately with warm water and a syringe. Don't dig into the ear with hard, sharp instruments. If the object is a button or other smooth, non-irritating substance, pull the flap of the ear outward, backward and upward and hold the head so that, with a little shaking, the object may roll out. If this fails, syringe the ear and it may be washed out. If this does not expel the object, do not worry. A little delay will do no harm, so take the patient to a doctor without trying to do anything further yourself.

Epistaxis (*Nose-Bleed*).—Some people have a great tendency to nose-bleed. In these people any little thing, such as sudden exercise, overheating or even unusual emotion, will start the bleeding. With other people, however, a nose-bleed is the result of a blow, or of picking or violently blowing the nose when it is inflamed. The bleeding usually comes from a point on the septum or middle piece of the nose, a very little distance back from the surface. Certain general disorders such as pneumonia, typhoid or some diseases of the heart, may begin with a nose-bleed.

TREATMENT.—An ordinary nose-bleed is easily stopped. Do not have the patient lie down unless he becomes very faint or dizzy. Place ice or cold cloths at the back of the neck and just under the nose, pressing hard against the upper lip. This will act reflexly, causing the artery to contract; direct pressure will close the artery. A very few moments of this pressure is enough to cause clotting of the blood. Then simply avoid blowing the nose, "hawking," or coughing, for some time.

If the bleeding continues, the nostril must be plugged. Unless a doctor is doing this, it is better not to use cotton, for you may not be able to get it all out. It is better to use linen or gauze bandage, taking care to push it in gently and always to keep an end of it out. The plug must be removed in twenty-four hours. As this sometimes starts bleeding, it must be done very gently and if possible by a doctor.

Foreign Bodies in the Nose.—Children are the only persons who are likely to have foreign bodies in their noses. They usually do not tell of it unless it hurts, and the first their parents know of it is when they notice a discharge from one side of the nose with a bad odor to it. It is not safe for any one but a doctor to attempt to remove such an object.

Acute Coryza, Catarrh of the Nose and Throat (*Cold in the Head*).—What is commonly called a "cold" in the head, throat or chest is really an infective inflammation of the mucous membrane, caused by a germ. The exposure of the patient to a draft or sudden chilling simply causes a lessened resistance and thus gives the germ a chance to develop.

Overheated houses, dressing too warmly in the house and not warmly enough out of doors, or failing to keep the feet dry and warm, are all important factors in starting a cold.

A daily cold bath, plenty of outdoor exercise and proper clothing are the most effective ways of avoiding a cold in the head.

SYMPTOMS.—A cold begins with a feeling of chilliness and sneezing. The nose at first feels dry; later, full of secretion. There may be headache and fever. It is at the first stage that treatment should be started or else it does very little good in shortening an attack.

TREATMENT.—The first and best thing to do is to open the bowels thoroughly with calomel and salts. This depletes the system of fluid also. Then take a hot lemonade and ten grains of quinine or a five-grain Dover's powder and go to bed, wrapping up warmly. This will give a good sweat and may entirely cure the cold.

After the secretions have begun to form in the nose, local applications are the only things of value. At first, a watery solution is best, sprayed in the nose. Later, an oily solution is better.

If babies have fever with their cold, 5 or 10 drops of sweet spirits of nitre may be given every two or three hours.

The "cold" sometimes extends down the throat, causing loss of voice. An ointment made up of oil of Wintergreen 2 drams, Lanolin 1 ounce, rubbed on the throat at night, and left under flannel until morning will relieve the loss of voice very promptly.

Another method of treatment is to take a quart or so of boiling hot water in a pitcher, add 2 drams (teaspoonfuls) of compound tincture of benzoin and inhale the hot vapor, both head and pitcher being wrapped in a towel.

Any extension into the lungs, causing cough and expectoration (spitting up) should cause one to send for a doctor immediately. Many an untended "cold" has turned into a bad bronchitis or consumption.

Thrush, Sprue (*Sore Mouth*).—Inflammation of the mouth may be of various kinds and variously produced. Uncleanliness is the most frequent cause. Irritation of a sharp tooth may start the condition. Mercury given in excess will cause a particularly severe form. Children are the most frequent sufferers. The symptoms are as follows:

Symptoms.—The mouth is hot, dry and painful. The child will not eat. The tongue is coated, the breath is bad, and later the child drools saliva copiously.

Treatment.—The simplest form requires very little treatment. Frequent rinsing of the mouth with boric acid solution; a cathartic, preferably castor oil; and the removal of the cause of the irritation, if it is a tooth, and the child will quickly be well again. Some antiseptic mouth-wash is very good.

Thrush or sprue is a more severe type of sore mouth, due to a special fungus. This forms in the mouth white flaky spots which look like curds of milk. There may also be with the disease, fever, vomiting and diarrhœa. In little babies, this disease is the result of unclean rubber nipples and nursing bottles. The latter should be thoroughly cleaned and boiled; the former should be cleaned and then kept in a boric acid solution. The child's mouth should be swabbed out with a solution of baking soda and water (a teaspoonful to a glass) every two or three hours.

If thrush is neglected, a child may develop ulcers in the mouth or actual spots of gangrene (decaying matter). The same condition may follow measles, scarlet fever or other severe illness. This is very serious, so that any mouth condition which does not clear up promptly should receive a doctor's care without delay.

Canker Sore.—This is a small, superficial ulcer which appears as a result of indigestion. Cure the indigestion and the canker heals readily. But as it is painful, anything that hurries the healing is welcome. Touch the canker with a stick of lunar caustic, taking care not to press too deeply nor to touch surrounding tissue. Then rinse the mouth in warm salt solution.

Acute Pharyngitis (*Mild Sore Throat*).—This is a congestion and irritation of the entire back of the throat. Acute indigestion, "cold" or exposure to wet and cold may bring it on. The throat is reddened, dry, hot, and there is an irritative throat cough which does not come from the lungs.

TREATMENT.—The treatment consists of gargling with any mild antiseptic, such as soda bicarbonate (a teaspoonful in a glass of water), a good cathartic, resting the throat by not talking, singing or smoking, and the patient is well.

Tonsilitis.—This is an inflammation of the tonsils. They become red, swollen and dotted with white spots, which are the follicles full of a cheesy material.

The general symptoms of a tonsilitis are severe. The fever is high, the pain is intense, so that the patient cannot eat, sleep or breathe with comfort. There is headache and backache. This condition is so much like diphtheria in some of its symptoms, that no unskilled person should trust himself to tell the difference between them. He should send for a doctor immediately.

TREATMENT.—The patient should be put to bed

and his dishes, etc., kept separate. This for two reasons: Because tonsilitis is infectious and because the disease may be diphtheria.

Give a good cathartic, let the patient have an ice-bag to hold against his throat, and let him have some gargle, such as has been mentioned above. The doctor, when he comes, will do whatever else is necessary.

Quinsy.—This is an abscess around the tonsils. It begins very much like tonsilitis, but the pain and difficulty in swallowing are greater. The glands of the neck become swollen, and the voice becomes inarticulate. It is a most painful and distressing sickness. In a few days the abscess forms and ruptures, when the patient is almost instantly better.

TREATMENT.—Antiseptic gargles and ice-bags to the throat first. With the first appearance of the abscess the doctor lances it, saving days of suffering.

Of course, keep the patient in bed, give a cathartic and cold, soft food.

In convalescence, the patient usually needs a tonic.

Toothache.—Unless there is a cavity in a tooth, there is little that a layman can do to ease the pain. If there is a cavity, clean it carefully and then pack cotton into it, first saturating it with oil of clove or wood creosote. Do not use any excess of the wood creosote, for it is poisonous if swallowed. See a dentist.

Alveolar Abscess (*Ulcerated Tooth*).—This begins in the socket of the tooth as an inflammation, and is excessively painful because of the unyielding character of the tissues. The pus cannot escape and hence causes great pressure. A dentist should be seen immediately, for prompt treatment may save the patient from having an abscess, or at least from having the nerve killed. The "ulcerated" tooth is tender on any pressure.

Mouth Breathing.—This is a condition due to adenoids, enlarged tonsils, or any obstructive growth in the nose. The patient, usually a child, breathes continually through the mouth, is apt to snore at night and is dull, stupid and in rather poor general health. Continuous breathing through the mouth is very bad for the child's lungs. The inspired air should be warmed and moistened by the nasal passages. When taken through the mouth, it is colder, drier and laden with the dust of the air. This is irritating to the throat and lungs, and productive of "colds," as well as laryngitis and bronchitis.

The quality of the voice is changed. Mouth

breathers have a whining voice, or as people generally say, they talk "through the nose."

TREATMENT.—The obstruction, whatever it is, adenoids, polyps of nose or enlarged bones of nose, should be removed by the surgeon as soon as possible. It is wonderful how quickly a sickly, puny child will become healthy and strong after such treatment. Of course, fresh air, good food and a tonic aid in this recovery. Do not wait too long before having these growths removed. A great deal of chronic deafness arises from adenoids which have been neglected.

CHAPTER IX

GENERAL DISEASES

Acute Articular Rheumatism (*Rheumatic Fever, Inflammatory Rheumatism*).—Certain factors seem necessary for the production of rheumatic fever. Some are—exposure to cold and wet, heredity, certain fevers and diseases; childbirth, lowered vitality and previous attacks. This form of rheumatism is rare before seven and after fifty years of age.

SYMPTOMS.—As a rule, the disease begins suddenly, generally at night. The patient has a chilly sensation, and severe pains, with stiffness of the joints. One joint may be affected, become almost normal after a few hours and then the disease may skip to another joint. The large joints, such as the knee, hip, shoulder or elbow are those usually attacked.

In children, a sore throat is often present, with pain under the chest bone.

Sometimes nausea and vomiting occur, followed by fever.

The sweating is excessive after the affection has begun, the thirst is great and constipation is the rule.

Only when the fever gets dangerously high is delirium present. The patient loses sleep on account of the pain and the sweating. Locally, there will be heat, tenderness, pain, swelling and redness of the skin about the joint affected.

In rheumatism, there is what is called the "Law of Parallelism." The joints affected are either all on one side of the body, or those on both sides are the same. The following seem to have an affinity: hip and shoulder, elbow and wrist, knee and ankle.

DURATION.—The duration of the disease varies. Some attacks, with careful treatment last only a few days; others may be prolonged for months, with all sorts of complications. When death occurs in an attack, it is usually due to the very high fever, lack of proper treatment or a condition of alcoholism in the patient.

TREATMENT.—In every case put the patient in bed. There must be absolute rest. Remove the sheets from the bed and wrap woolen cloths or blankets about the patient, being careful to protect the inflamed joint from the weight of the coverings. The diet should be mild. Milk is the best food and plenty of water should be given; especially the alkaline mineral waters. The affected joint may be rubbed with oil of wintergreen, and wrapped in cotton-wool or flannel and soaked with the following:

Oil of Wintergreen.........1 ounce
Compound soap liniment...8 ounces

Chronic Articular Rheumatism.—The chronic form is an affection characterized by pain and stiffness of the joints, but the onset is not sudden, and there is no fever or sweating. It occurs after middle life; is observed usually in the poor and is markedly influenced by changes of temperature. The victims of this disorder make excellent weather prophets.

Symptoms.—The main symptoms are aching pains in one or more joints, generally the knees or ankles. The joint is a little tender and swollen, the pain growing worse at night and after sitting still all day. There is no fever. The muscles and tissues about the joint shrink, causing the joint to appear swollen.

The prospect of complete recovery is not good after the middle of life, but the disease does not affect the duration of life unless by interfering with exercise and sleep.

Treatment.—The symptoms may be relieved to

a great extent, by drugs, prescribed by a physician, but there is no curative treatment.

Turkish and Russian baths, massage, local douches and electricity are all employed with more or less success. Liniments and ointments may also be employed; and all people who suffer with rheumatism should wear flannel underclothing. Woolen knee-caps sometimes prove beneficial.

Muscular Rheumatism.—This is a rheumatic condition of the muscles of the body.

SYMPTOMS.—As a rule, the first attack is very acute and its onset sudden with pain, slight tenderness, and stiffness of the muscles involved. The pain, tenderness, and stiffness are increased by any attempt at movement. These symptoms may be constant or they may only be brought out on motion. Fever is absent and there are no local signs.

The acute variety seldom lasts more than six or eight days, while the chronic form recurs frequently with atmospheric changes, and may become constant. Some of the muscles affected are those of the head, giving pain on both sides of the head, aggravated by movements of the muscles; those of the eye which may be affected so that moving the eye causes pain: and the muscles of the lower jaw.

When the neck muscles are involved, wry or stiff neck results. The attack is generally limited to one side of the neck, toward which the head is twisted, and great pain is experienced when one attempts to move the head to the other side.

This form of rheumatism may affect the muscles of the chest, giving rise to a condition that is sometimes mistaken for pleurisy. Pain is caused by forced breathing, coughing and sneezing.

It may also affect the muscles of the lower back; this is the most common variety. It is commonly called lumbago. Both sides are usually affected. It is sometimes associated with acute sciatica, when the pain is agonizing.

This condition is not dangerous to life. The attacks may be relieved by prompt and proper treatment by a physician, but the rheumatic tendency is often hard to eradicate.

Treatment.—Put the patient to bed in order to insure absolute rest. If the chest muscles are affected, firmly strap the affected side with broad strips of adhesive plaster, extending from the backbone to the chest-bone.

A poultice of flax-seed meal, changed every one to three hours, is successful in many acute cases.

The bowels should be kept open. Salts are the best means to accomplish this. Massage, hot-air baths, and electricity are all measures that have some value.

Arthritis Deformans (*Rheumatic Gout*).—This is a destructive disease of the joints, attended by bony formations about the articulations, causing a loss of motion and deformity.

The cause of this trouble is very doubtful. It occurs most frequently in women past middle life. Among some of the so-called causes may be mentioned—unhealthful living, exposure, injury, frequent child-births, change of life, grief, mental worry, tuberculosis, heredity and frequent attacks of acute articular rheumatism.

SYMPTOMS.—This disease may either be acute or chronic.

Acute.—Several joints are attacked at the same time and slight fever may be present. The involved joints are swollen and painful; but there is no heat or redness present. The attack subsides more or less to recur after a varying interval.

Chronic.—In this form only one joint at first is attacked as a rule. The joints of the fingers are mostly the ones involved in the beginning. The joint gradually becomes swollen and painful, the pain being caused or made worse by any attempt at movement.

As the disease advances, the wrists, ankles,

elbows, knees, jaws, and spine are involved. The corresponding joints on each side of the body are affected simultaneously. Movement becomes difficult and in a short time the joints become rigid. The muscles waste away.

The fingers are bent toward the palm and drawn to the "little-finger" side of the hand.

The patient lies with the thighs and legs drawn up.

In addition to the pain there may be tingling, numbness, local sweating and a discoloration of the skin.

This disease is slow, and gradually involves all the joints, rendering the patient a helpless invalid.

If early treatment is established, the disease may be held in check for several years. Otherwise it is incurable, although it may make no advances for a long time.

TREATMENT.—The diet should be carefully selected and the general hygiene receive attention. Employ all measures to improve the general health.

Early in the disease the joints may be rubbed with cod-liver oil; and internally, effervescing lithium citrate, a teaspoonful three times a day is beneficial.

Gout.—Gout is a disorder of nutrition with a

disturbance between the building up and breaking down processes of the body, and an excess of uric acid in the blood.

SYMPTOMS.—Acute gout is comparatively rare in the United States. Chronic gout results from a repetition of acute attacks. Before the attack there are troubles of digestion; namely, acidity, flatulence, loss of appetite, constipation, and scanty, highly colored urine.

The joint affection is often slow in developing and a good deal of minor uneasiness in the part may be for some time complained of, before the actual symptoms appear. The ball of the great toe (sometimes the ankle, heel or instep) at first feels somewhat hot and painful, and the pain increases quickly in severity until it becomes intense and almost unbearable; the tenderness is also exquisite, and the patient cannot endure even the contact of the bed clothes. There is some chilliness, followed by fever. The pain after a few hours is less severe. The veins around the painful joint first appear swollen and shortly the whole joint becomes swollen, tense, shiny and of a deep red color. For the next few days there will be an increase in the fever and other symptoms during the evening and a decrease in the morning.

It is not uncommon for the other foot to be attacked in precisely the same manner.

The duration of the attack is variable; it may be over in a few days, or there may be a series of minor attacks which may incapacitate the patient for many weeks.

TREATMENT.—In the acute variety, the family will get a physician because they will be impressed with the severity of the symptoms. All that can be done is to make the patient comfortable until the doctor arrives.

In the chronic forms the diet, habits, mode of living, etc., should be subjected to regulation.

The patient should be forbidden to indulge in pastry, hot bread, cakes, sweetmeats, spices, condiments, veal, liver, mutton, beef, lamb, pork, cheese, tomatoes, beans, oatmeal, sugar, tea, coffee, wines, and malt liquors.

The proper foods are: milk, butter, oysters, fish, vegetables (except as above), and fruits, except strawberries, lemons and oranges.

Drink water freely, especially the alkaline waters.

Effervescing citrate of lithia, one teaspoonful in water three times a day, and the saline laxatives.

The underclothing should be woolen and if possible a warm climate is advised.

Exercise, massage, cold bathing, Turkish baths, etc., cautiously employed, are of great benefit.

Diabetes Mellitus.—Diabetes Mellitus is a chronic affection, characterized by the constant presence of sugar in the urine, an excessive urinary discharge, and the progressive loss of flesh and weight.

Causes.—It occurs usually in the male sex, between the ages of twenty-five and fifty years. It is rare in the Negro race.

Some of the important causative factors are heredity, disorders of the nervous and urinary systems, excessive use of farinaceous foods, malt liquors and mental anxiety.

Symptoms.—The symptoms in different individuals having diabetes differ, both as to their course and severity. A typical case is the following:

There is a sweetish taste in the mouth; and the saliva is acid, which soon destroys the teeth. The mouth and throat are dry, giving rise to great thirst. With the progressive emaciation there is great increase of appetite. Constipation is the rule. The skin is usually dry and harsh. Boils are frequent. The patient is nervous and irritable, there is eye trouble and cataracts may appear. The constitutional disturbances are overwhelming. The urine is increased to three or four quarts a day.

In young people, the disease may be fatal in five weeks or in half a year. The older the patient when the disease first appears, the longer he is likely to live.

TREATMENT.—If the above symptoms are present, a physician should be sought, in order that he may examine the urine and make a positive diagnosis.

The treatment is mostly dietetic, cutting out the main starchy foods, but this should not be carried too far at the expense of the general health.

The patient should eat meats of every kind, soups made with meat and without flour; game, poultry, fish, oysters, lobsters, crabs, eggs, butter, cheese, oils, fats, cream, butter-milk, spinach, celery, lettuce, cabbage, tomatoes, asparagus tops, water-cress, string beans, onions, cucumbers, pickles, olives, unsweetened jellies, tea and coffee without sugar, carbonated waters, and bread made from gluten, bran or almond flour.

The foods that should not be eaten are: ordinary bread or flour, sugar, honey, potatoes, parsnips, peas, barley, beans, rice, tapioca, arrowroot, cracked wheat, oatmeal, turnips, beets, corn, carrots, prunes, grapes, figs, bananas, pears, peaches, watermelons, cantaloupes, chestnuts, chocolate,

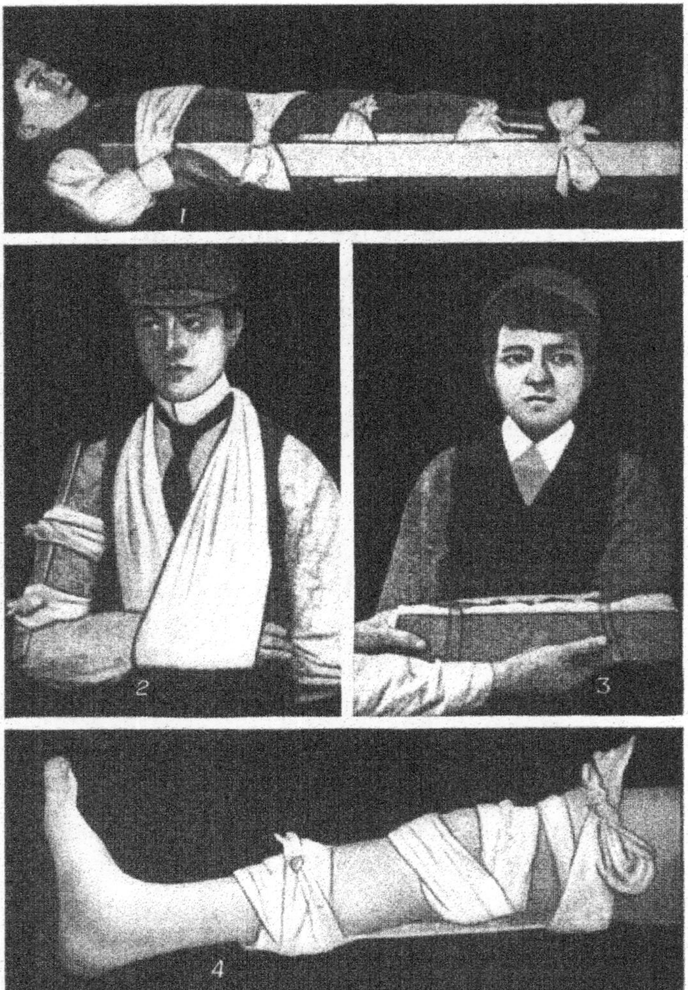

1. EMERGENCY SPLINT FOR A BROKEN LEG
2. EMERGENCY SPLINT FOR A BROKEN UPPER ARM
3. EMERGENCY SPLINT FOR A BROKEN FOREARM
4. EMERGENCY SPLINT FOR A BROKEN KNEEPAN

biscuits, pastry, syrups, preserves, sweet wines, and malt liquors.

When the patient wishes to sweeten the food, saccharin or glycerin may be used.

The hygienic treatment is important. Fresh air, daily bathing, and exercise should be regularly indulged in. The exercise should be regulated according to the patient's strength. Avoid over-exertion. The underclothing should be made of flannel.

Most drugs recommended for this condition are useless, but a competent physician can prescribe certain medicines that will materially aid the general health of the patient.

CHAPTER X

DISEASES OF THE BLOOD AND HEART

Normal blood is made up principally of solid bodies (called corpuscles) and a fluid called serum. There are two kinds of blood-corpuscles, namely, red and white. The red corpuscles vary in number from 4,500,000 to 5,000,000 to the cubic millimeter. The red corpuscles contain what is called "hemoglobin," which carries the oxygen of the blood. The white blood-cells number from 7,000 to 10,000 to the cubic millimeter.

The color of the blood is not constant. To the naked eye, the blood from an artery is of a bright red color, while blood from a vein is darker in color. If the oxygen supply is interfered with from any cause, the blood becomes darker.

Certain blood diseases and poisons change the color of the blood. When the quality of the blood is changed or the normal proportion of the red and white cells is interfered with, the result is a blood disease.

When a person has a blood disease, there are present certain symptoms that give a clue to the diagnosis. But, to be accurate, an examination of the blood must be made. The treatment of all diseases of the blood is hygienic and medicinal. Therefore, in order to have a positive diagnosis made and the proper treatment instituted, a competent physician should be consulted.

Anemia.—Anemia is a lessening in the number of red blood corpuscles or of the entire quantity of the blood.

CAUSES.—The female is very liable to anemia. It occurs often in women who are pregnant or nearing the age when change of life occurs.

Poor or insufficient quantity of food will cause anemia. Other causes are lack of air or sunshine, prolonged labor with mental worry, prolonged nursing, bleeding, Bright's Disease, malaria, cancer and certain poisons.

SYMPTOMS.—The patient has a pale and pallid look. Even the mucous membranes, inside the mouth, inside the eyelid, etc., are affected.

Weakness and loss of strength are noticed.

The appetite is lost, the digestion of food is faulty and vomiting sometimes occurs. At times there may be a slight fever.

There are certain mental symptoms present,

varying in degree, according to the severity of the disease. They are: irritability, swooning, fainting fits and hysteria.

The ankles often swell. When this swelling is pressed it shows a pitting that lasts, sometimes, for several minutes. This condition is called edema.

The patient complains of shortness of breath and palpitation of the heart.

OUTCOME.—In this disease, if the cause is discovered early enough, if no complications are present, and treatment is started, the outcome is favorable.

TREATMENT.—Rest is essential. All forms of exercise should be restricted. Fresh air, sunlight, and a diet that is highly nutritious are advised.

Avoid constipation by taking salts or the laxative mineral waters.

For the various tonics required in this disease, a physician should be seen.

Chlorosis (*Green Sickness*).—This is a pronounced anemia, common mostly to girls about the age of puberty.

CAUSES.—Some of the causes of green sickness are said to be overwork, bad air and food, menstrual disorders, emotional disturbances and a change of climate. Society girls who keep late hours are liable to this disease. It occurs most often in cities.

Green sickness may continue up to twenty-four years of age with recurrences. A mother with a tuberculous tendency may have a daughter with chlorosis.

SYMPTOMS.—As a rule, a disorder in menstruation is first noticed, such as an irregularity or suppression of the menstruation or an excessive menstrual flow. Shortly after this condition is observed, the complexion changes. This change, as a rule, is uniform and characteristic. Blondes become pale and waxy-looking. The face also looks puffy. Brunettes become "muddy-looking" and black rings appear under the eyes.

Upon the slightest exertion fatigue results. Shortness of breath is common.

The disposition of the individual changes. He becomes morose and melancholy and suffers from attacks of hysteria.

The appetite is perverted and the digestion impaired.

Strange to say, there is no loss of flesh. In fact, the patient appears stout.

After a time the skin assumes a characteristic yellowish-green tinge.

Headaches and neuralgia may be present.

Constipation accompanies most cases.

OUTCOME.—Death from this disease is rare. Chlorosis is a chronic trouble, subject to relapses and complications.

TREATMENT.—The most important factor in the treatment of this disease is the consideration of the hygiene of the patient. The surroundings should be pleasant and healthful. The quality of the food should be improved.

The patient should live out of doors in the sunshine and do little or no work.

For the constipation, saline laxatives and mineral waters are advised.

In severe cases the patient should rest in bed.

The blood should be examined from time to time in order to know the effect of the treatment.

Hemophilia (*Bleeders' Disease*).—This is a condition characterized by a tendency to uncontrollable bleeding with or without abrasions.

CAUSE.—The most important cause is heredity. The male sex is most affected.

SYMPTOMS.—In nearly every case, bleeding occurs about the time the child is cutting its teeth.

Spontaneous bleeding happens from the membranes of the nose, mouth, lungs, stomach and intestines.

In typical cases, there is bleeding from the

fingers, toes, lobes of the ears, backs of the hands and arms, without any apparent changes in the skin.

This bleeding will continue for days and weeks in spite of all treatment.

Bleeding from the nose is common.

Outcome.—In many cases this disease ends fatally. Death never occurs, however, during the first bleeding. The younger the person when the disease begins, the more serious the result. Sometimes the patient outgrows the tendency to bleeding.

Treatment.—Very little can be done for this affection.

Locally, at the time of bleeding, pressure, ice, heat, tannic or gallic acid may be used. In every case a physician should be consulted.

Scorbutus (*Scurvy*).—Scurvy is a peculiar condition due to improper nourishment.

Causes.—The most important cause is the lack of fresh vegetables in the diet. Unhygienic surroundings added to this fault of diet, aid the condition. It occurs most frequently in sailors, especially those who go on long trips, on sailing vessels, in men's prisons and armies; in fact, among men collected in numbers under unhygienic conditions.

SYMPTOMS.—The onset of scurvy is slow. The person affected first notices that he is weak, feels lazy, has fits of mental depression and is anemic.

The skin becomes rough, dry and muddy looking. The face looks pale and bloated.

The main symptoms are referred to the gums. They become swollen and spongy with a tendency to bleed on the slightest provocation. The teeth may loosen and fall out.

The breath becomes offensive.

The eyes appear sunken and dark circles appear under them.

Minute points of bleeding from the skin are common.

Pain, tenderness and swelling of the joints, disturbances of sight and constipation may occur.

OUTCOME.—Recovery is the rule with early and proper treatment.

TREATMENT.—To be successful in treating this disease, two main points must be remembered:

First: Remove the patient to sanitary quarters.

Second: Give plenty of fresh vegetables and fruits.

Some of the foods that are beneficial in this condition are raw cabbage, cresses, potatoes, sauerkraut, onions, lemon juice, oranges and acid fruits.

Added to this diet should be fresh meats, milk and fish.

Give salines for constipation if needed.

In all forms keep the mouth clean with antiseptic solutions.

Heart Disease.—The term "heart disease" is indefinite. There are several heart lesions, each one a disease in itself. It would be impracticable here to discuss the pathological conditions of the heart, but the objective signs of heart trouble will be described, and the general term, "Heart Disease," used.

CAUSES.—Many factors give rise to this trouble. Sometimes a person is born with a heart which is not normal. Very often that organ is affected by other diseases, and not infrequently the individual brings heart trouble upon himself by some unhealthy course of living.

When heart disease is congenital the outlook is bad. As a rule, the person affected never becomes healthy and robust, but lives the life of a chronic invalid, always under the care of a physician or of parents who have been instructed regarding the dangers of the malady.

When an abnormal heart condition results from disease, much can be done to repair the damage.

Some of the various diseases that affect the

heart are rheumatism, influenza, scarlet fever, smallpox, puerperal fever, Bright's Disease, gout, scurvy, anemia, diabetes, pneumonia, erysipelas, meningitis, chorea, syphilis, and some other diseases.

The heart may be injured by prolonged and violent muscular exertion, and by the prolonged use of stimulants, such as alcohol, tobacco, tea and coffee.

SYMPTOMS.—The signs of a diseased heart condition are:

Dropsy.—This is a filling up by serum of the cavities and tissues of the body. It is indicative of heart disease, especially when it affects both sides of the body.

When dropsy is localized in certain regions, as the ankles, it is termed *edema*. When it is generalized it is known as *anasarca*. These are serious signs and should not be taken lightly by either the patient or his friends.

When there is a disturbance of the general circulation and the oxidation of the blood is deficient, the body surface becomes blue. This is called *cyanosis*. It accompanies various forms of chronic heart disease.

Pain in the region of the heart may be due to any one of several things. It may be caused by a disease of the covering of the heart (the pericardium), by neuralgia, localized pleurisy, bone disease, or abscess. Heart disease may give rise to exquisite pain in the stomach.

Valvular disease and angina pectoris (see Angina Pectoris) cause pain in the heart.

Dyspnœa, or difficult breathing, is a sign of heart disease and may be caused by exertion, or it may occur paroxysmally.

Heart disease may cause brain symptoms, such as vertigo, faintness, dullness, languor, moderate delirium, coma, chorea, epileptic form of convulsions, etc.

Attending heart disease may be disorders of indigestion, such as dyspepsia, flatulence, nausea and vomiting.

When there is an inability to breathe except in the upright position; when a dry, hacking cough is present; also headache, restlessness and delirium of varying degrees, a diseased heart condition will probably be found.

A rapid heart may be normal to the individual or may show an abnormal condition.

The heart beat is normally accelerated by physical or mental exertion, fear, excitement, pleasure, etc., by a heavy meal, or when the erect posture is assumed.

When accelerated abnormally the cause may be drugs, fevers, heart disease, reflex irritation, goiter or various brain conditions.

Very often the heart beats faster than is normal to the individual and no cause can be discovered.

An infrequency of the heart (slow heart) may be normal or due to jaundice, hardening of the arteries, heart disease, drugs or brain conditions.

DIAGNOSIS.—Unskilled persons are not expected to make a diagnosis. There are conditions of the heart which only the most skilful physician can detect. When any of the obvious signs are present there should be no delay in calling a doctor. The objective symptoms taken collectively only point to a condition that may be present. A physical examination and a continued clinical study of the case, make a positive diagnosis.

OUTCOME.—As a rule, tell a man he has heart disease and he at once considers it fatal. This is not so. Many heart troubles can be absolutely cured; many can be improved by proper treatment, so that the patient can enjoy the work and pleasures of life. The underlying causes should be treated and made normal, and then the heart will become normal. Some heart conditions end fatally, and when a diseased condition is suspected, call a physician and leave the case to him.

TREATMENT.—Rest is of value in all cardiac conditions. Under some circumstances rest is indispensable.

In all cases, the individual should be warned against great physical exertion, such as athletic work, rapid walking, running, going up stairs quickly, and excessive exercise of any kind.

He should guard against the extremes of passion, exposure to cold and wet and irregular living.

The diet should be nourishing but bland. Do not overwork the stomach. Eat moderately of plain, wholesome food.

All stimulants, such as liquors, tobacco, tea and coffee, should be forbidden.

Observe all the rules of hygiene.

The bowels should be kept in action, using, if needed, laxatives or purgatives.

Some doctors advise passive exercise and massage and baths; but this question, as well as the medicines necessary for the particular form of heart disease present should be left to the physician selected by the patient.

Angina Pectoris (*Neuralgia of the Heart, Breast Pang*).—Attacks of sharp heart pains, extending usually to the left shoulder and down the left arm, accompanied by a feeling of constriction of the chest and a terrifying fear of impending death.

Causes.—The tendency may be inherited. Syphilis and hysteria may exert an influence in causing the disease. The main cause is poor nutrition of the heart, causing temporary inability of the heart to do its work. Males after forty years of age are most affected. The attacks are precipitated by sudden strain, particularly after meals, great mental excitement or acute indigestion. Cold will bring on an attack; also constipation and pressure from the accumulation of gas.

Symptoms.—Pain, beginning in the heart and extending to the neck and down the left arm is the chief sign of this disease.

The chest is fixed and there is shortness of breath. The face is pale, anxious and covered with drops of sweat. There is a horrifying fear of death.

The pain lasts only a few seconds or minutes, and while death does not occur, the attack is followed by extreme prostration.

A cessation of the pain ends the attack. It is followed by vomiting and the passing of a large amount of urine.

These attacks bring about a mental change. The sufferer becomes gloomy, suicidal, and sometimes develops epilepsy.

There is a false variety of angina pectoris which is common with nervous women and children and some men. This form comes on gradually. The symptoms are distention of the abdomen, eructation of gases, great nervousness, flushed face, diffused heart pain and general hysterical signs.

OUTCOME.—The first attack of genuine angina pectoris may end in death, or the patient may have several attacks at varying periods, sometimes extending over years.

In the false variety the outcome is always good.

TREATMENT.—During the attack there is little to be done. If within reach of a drug-store, get some pearls of amyl nitrite and break them in a handkerchief. Let the patient inhale the fumes from the handkerchief. Chronic sufferers always carry these with them. During the interval between the attacks, an attempt should be made to correct the underlying causes or to lessen their influence.

The diet should be selected so that flatulency and constipation do not occur.

Avoid mental excitement and physical exertion.

Tonics are of great value in these cases. Hot baths may be of benefit.

Never permit *cold baths,* for they are positively *harmful.*

The false variety requires the same treatment as hysteria.

Arteriosclerosis (***Hardening of the Arteries***). —This is a chronic, degenerative and inflammatory disease of the blood vessels, resulting in an overgrowth of the tissues of the arteries, followed by chalky deposits. The changes may extend to the capillaries and veins.

This condition causes an impairment of the arterial circulation, together with a degeneration in other organs and an impairment of their nutrition.

CAUSES.—The main causes are old age, heredity, alcoholism, syphilis, lead poisoning, exposure and excesses of various kinds.

The saying is, "A man is as old as his arteries."

SYMPTOMS.—Very often no signs are present except the "pipe-stem" feeling of the arteries.

When the arteries of the brain are affected there may be attacks of fainting, false apoplectic attacks or spells of unconsciousness. Hardening of the arteries in any of the organs, gives rise to trouble in the organ thus affected.

OUTCOME.—The condition may be prevented or held in check, but cannot be removed. Life may be terminated by a stroke of apoplexy, heart failure or by a kidney lesion.

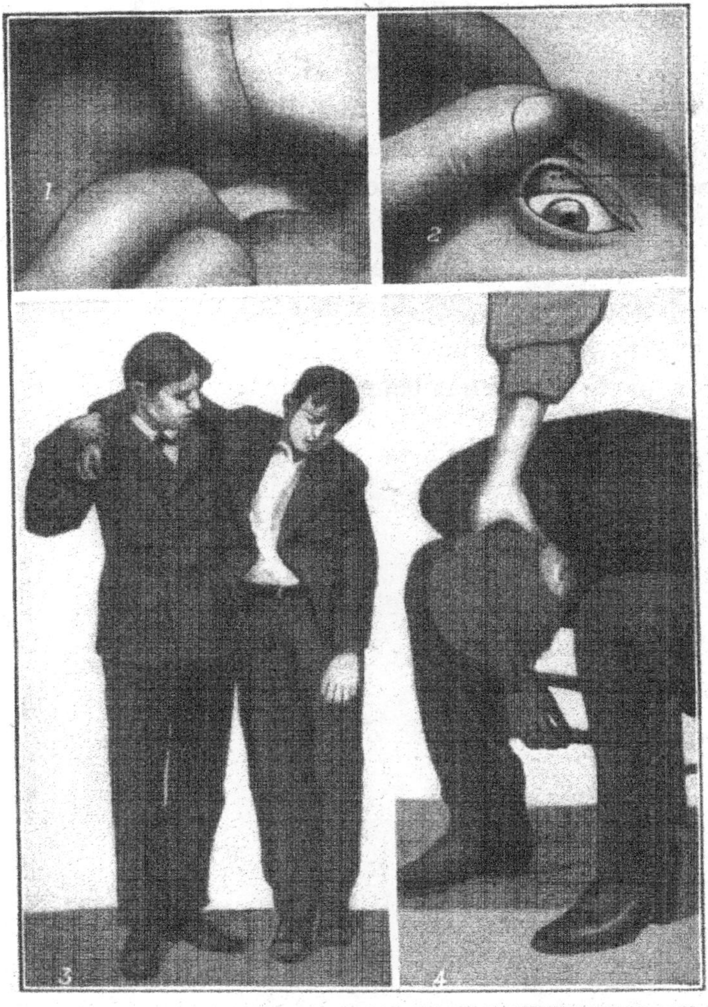

1 AND 2. REMOVING CINDER FROM EYE. THE LID IS FIRST PULLED DOWN AS IN 1, AND THEN WITH THE OTHER FINGER AGAINST IT, IS TURNED WRONG SIDE OUT AS IN 2

3. METHOD OF SUPPORTING A PERSON WHO IS FAINT

4. POSITION TO PLACE A FAINTING PERSON IN. THE HEAD WELL DOWN BRINGS THE BLOOD BACK TO THE BRAIN

TREATMENT.—The habits of living should be regular and without excesses, and the diet should be chosen with care. If the cause or causes are known they should be removed. Alcohol, tea and coffee are very harmful in these cases.

Constipation should be avoided. Keep the bowels freely open. Eat few meats. Drink plenty of water.

Moderate exercise is beneficial.

CHAPTER XI

DISEASES OF THE KIDNEYS AND BLADDER

Most people use one term for all forms of nephritis, namely, Bright's Disease, and the technical medical name need not be given here.

Chronic Bright's Disease has several varieties, but the symptoms for all forms are, in the main, similar. The positive diagnosis is made by a laboratory examination of the urine. Therefore, it is essential to have a physician in attendance, in order to take specimens of urine, and also to treat the disease, any form of which is very dangerous to the health and life of the individual.

Acute uremia or uremic poisoning or uremic convulsions are a group of nervous phenomena, which may develop during the course of either acute or chronic Bright's Disease, or other maladies, the result of the retention or accumulation in the blood of poisonous material. This condition is very serious and often terminates in death.

Acute Bright's Disease.—

CAUSES.—Acute Bright's Disease may be caused by exposure to cold and wet, scarlet fever, diphtheria, malaria, and other infectious diseases, injury to the back, pregnancy and the continued use of irritants, such as turpentine, Spanish fly, phosphorus, ginger, etc. It may also be associated with certain skin diseases, large burns of the skin and simple tonsilitis. This disease is most common in children.

SYMPTOMS.—As a rule, it begins suddenly with nausea, violent vomiting, fever and a dull pain over the kidneys, radiating down the back. The patient experiences a desire to urinate frequently, but can pass only small quantities of urine, suffers from diarrhœa and the skin is harsh and dry.

In mild cases, dropsy develops slowly, the individual becomes anemic and has shortness of breath. He feels very much weakened. The dropsy begins first in the eyelids and the face, giving an appearance of puffiness. Later it becomes generalized.

Acute Bright's Disease lasts from one to four weeks.

OUTCOME.—The outcome is generally good, recovery occurring in many cases when the treatment is prompt and appropriate. Uremic convulsions may, however, occur and lead to death. It may pass into chronic Bright's Disease.

Treatment.—Put the patient to bed and keep him there until all the symptoms have disappeared. The ideal diet is milk, but if the weakness is marked, broths and even oysters may be allowed; also water or cream of tartar lemonade.

All stimulants—tea, coffee, beef tea and extracts—are prohibited. Call a doctor.

Chronic Bright's Disease. (a.) (*Large White Kidney.*)—

Causes.—Very rarely does it follow an acute attack. Young adults are for the most part the ones attacked; it is seldom observed after forty years of age.

Habitual exposure to cold and wet, malaria, syphilis, alcoholic excesses, lead poisoning, opium habit, tuberculosis and pregnancy are some of the principal causes.

Symptoms.—This disease begins slowly and takes hold of the individual before he is aware of his condition. He suffers from general ill health, anemia, disturbances of digestion, general weakness, puffiness about the eyes, most noticeable in the morning, shortness of breath and palpitation of the heart. After a while he vomits from no apparent cause, suffers from headaches, is troubled with fainting, or with defective vision and more or less generalized dropsy. Transient blindness may occur in the early stages, while permanent blindness is not uncommon late in the course of the disease. Anemia is very pronounced. Irritability of the bladder is a constant symptom, occurring early in the disease.

OUTCOME.—Severe cases may end in death within a few months or two years, while in milder cases, under skilful treatment, the patient may live an indefinite period.

(b.) Contracted Kidney (*Small Red Kidney, Gouty Kidney*).—This form of chronic Bright's Disease occurs usually in males from forty to sixty years of age.

CAUSES.—Some of the principal causes are gout, chronic lead poisoning, syphilis, alcoholism, opium habit, chronic inflammation of the bladder, chronic gonorrhœa, long, continued worry, anxiety or grief and hereditary influences.

SYMPTOMS.—In the majority of cases there are no characteristic early symptoms. The onset of the disease is insidious. The signs to attract attention are frequent urination, no dropsy, but a slight puffiness of the eyelids. Disorders of the sight occur frequently.

There is weakness, loss of weight, the skin is

dry and there is shortness of breath on exertion. Progressive anemia is a common sign.

Toward the end the urine diminishes in amount.

The duration is indefinite and the disease ends usually in death from convulsions and coma. It is essentially chronic, and cases have lasted as long as eleven years.

(c.) Amyloid Kidney (*Waxy Kidney*).—This variety of chronic Bright's Disease is caused chiefly by prolonged pus in the kidney or the bones, syphilis, cancer and consumption.

SYMPTOMS.—There are always symptoms of the underlying cause present. Together with these symptoms there may be swelling of the ankles, feet and legs, dropsy of the abdomen, and an increased flow of pale, watery urine.

OUTCOME.—If the disease causing the waxy kidney can be treated and cured before too much damage has been done the disease may be arrested, otherwise the outlook is discouraging.

TREATMENT OF CHRONIC BRIGHT'S DISEASE.—The first points to remember are: Put the patient to bed or keep him seated in a chair. Rest is most essential. The underclothing should be woolen. If possible, remove to a dry, warm climate. The diet is of great importance. Nitrogenous foods should be reduced to a minimum.

Milk may constitute the diet, pure, or prepared in various dishes, or the diet may be exclusively of lean meat, prepared by chopping it fine, removing all fibrous and fatty portions, boiling it quickly, salting to taste, and serving it hot. So-called "Salisbury steak" may be combined with the milk.

A half-pint of hot water, acidulated with the juice of half a lemon, may be taken before each meal to advantage.

Vegetables, chicken broth and eggs, soft boiled or poached in milk, may be tried.

All forms of alcoholic stimulation should be avoided.

A daily warm or hot bath is valuable, but never allow cold or sea bathing.

Regularity in the bowel movements is necessary, and to produce this the alkaline mineral waters, salts or cascara in the form of the fluid extract, a teaspoonful or two at night time, should be taken.

For the medicinal treatment and the treatment of the primary causes a doctor should be consulted in all cases.

(d.) Pyelitis (*Pus in the Urine, Suppurative Nephritis*).—

Causes.—The causes of this condition are exposure to cold and wet, inflammation of the blad-

Between the attacks there is more or less pain, with tenderness over the kidneys and the urine is stained with blood.

The X-rays should be employed in all cases to make a positive diagnosis. Therefore it is necessary to see a physician.

OUTCOME.—The outcome is favorable unless complications occur. Recurrences are common. The condition known as gravel is less dangerous than a case of calculus. If the stone is a large one, or if there are more than one, the outcome becomes proportionately more grave.

TREATMENT.—During the attack the object is to relieve the pain. A physician will be needed to prescribe the necessary drugs. While waiting for him a hot bath will do much to ease the suffering. Hot poultices and hot fomentations applied over the kidneys will afford some relief. Give water to drink freely.

A surgical operation may be necessary in order to remove the stone, if it is large and impacted or threatens the life of the patient.

Between the attacks the aim is to prevent the formation of the calculi. There are no remedies that will dissolve fully formed calculi, but there are ways by which the crystals of the blood and urine may be kept in solution, thus checking the formation of concretions. The alkaline waters are beneficial.

The diet should consist of milk and vegetables and a small quantity of meat.

As there are different forms of calculi and as the diet differs with some of the different forms, it is well to have an examination made to determine the variety, in order that the proper diet may be prescribed.

Acute Uremia, Uremic Coma or Convulsions.—"Uremic intoxication is the result of the failure of the kidneys to perform their normal function of eliminating some or all of the poisonous elements of the urine."—(From Hughes' *Practice of Medicine.*)

CAUSES.—This condition is caused by a suppression of urine, either from the acute or chronic form of Bright's Disease, from a cystic, tubercular, or cancerous kidney, the puerperal state, and operations on the uterus, bladder, urethra or rectum.

SYMPTOMS.—The acute outbreak may show itself in three ways, as the gastro-intestinal variety, convulsive variety and the cerebral variety or uremic coma.

(a.) Gastro-Intestinal Variety.—The patient has sudden fainting spells, becomes pale and nauseated, vomits and a fever appears. Convulsions der, cystitis, obstruction of the tubes leading from the kidneys to the bladder, pressure from a tumor, use of irritative drugs and certain infectious diseases.

Symptoms.—This disease often begins with chills and fever, shooting pains down the back and frequent urination.

The urine is milky in appearance when voided and deposits a large whitish or yellowish white sediment.

The formation of pus is indicated by chills, irregular fever sweats, pains over the kidneys and tenderness in the back.

In severe cases there may be low, muttering delirium, fissured and dry tongue, anemia, emaciation, stupor and coma.

Outcome.—Simple causes, in which there is no obstruction to the discharge, recover as a rule in a week or ten days. Otherwise the outcome is grave.

Treatment.—Put the patient to bed and confine the diet to milk. Give mineral alkaline waters freely.

Local applications of heat to the back will relieve the pain.

As suppuration is likely to supervene at any time a surgeon should be consulted early, for a prompt operation may save otherwise hopeless cases.

Renal Colic, Renal Calculi (*Gravel*).—By gravel is meant very small concretions (sand) which are often passed freely in the urine. Gravel may be discovered at all ages, but is most frequent in people from forty to fifty years of age.

The precise cause is not yet known.

Renal calculi are the larger stones which usually form in the kidney. When these stones get into the slender duct called the ureter, which leads from the kidney, and attempt to pass down the ureter, *renal colic* results.

SYMPTOMS.—Pain is the cardinal sign of renal calculi. It is an agonizing pain in the back, made worse by motion. The bladder is irritable, the face pallid and the features pinched.

Nausea and vomiting are sometimes present during the attack, as well as a subnormal surface temperature and faintness, but rarely unconsciousness.

The attack ends suddenly, the stone escaping into the bladder.

If the stone is not passed the attack may subside and begin again in a short time.

The urine usually escapes in drops and is stained with blood.

Between the attacks there is more or less pain, with tenderness over the kidneys and the urine is stained with blood.

The X-rays should be employed in all cases to make a positive diagnosis. Therefore it is necessary to see a physician.

Outcome.—The outcome is favorable unless complications occur. Recurrences are common. The condition known as gravel is less dangerous than a case of calculus. If the stone is a large one, or if there are more than one, the outcome becomes proportionately more grave.

Treatment.—During the attack the object is to relieve the pain. A physician will be needed to prescribe the necessary drugs. While waiting for him a hot bath will do much to ease the suffering. Hot poultices and hot fomentations applied over the kidneys will afford some relief. Give water to drink freely.

A surgical operation may be necessary in order to remove the stone, if it is large and impacted or threatens the life of the patient.

Between the attacks the aim is to prevent the formation of the calculi. There are no remedies that will dissolve fully formed calculi, but there are ways by which the crystals of the blood and urine may be kept in solution, thus checking the formation of concretions. The alkaline waters are beneficial.

The diet should consist of milk and vegetables and a small quantity of meat.

As there are different forms of calculi and as the diet differs with some of the different forms, it is well to have an examination made to determine the variety, in order that the proper diet may be prescribed.

Acute Uremia, Uremic Coma or Convulsions.—"Uremic intoxication is the result of the failure of the kidneys to perform their normal function of eliminating some or all of the poisonous elements of the urine."—(From Hughes' *Practice of Medicine.*)

CAUSES.—This condition is caused by a suppression of urine, either from the acute or chronic form of Bright's Disease, from a cystic, tubercular, or cancerous kidney, the puerperal state, and operations on the uterus, bladder, urethra or rectum.

SYMPTOMS.—The acute outbreak may show itself in three ways, as the gastro-intestinal variety, convulsive variety and the cerebral variety or uremic coma.

(a.) Gastro-Intestinal Variety.—The patient has sudden fainting spells, becomes pale and nauseated, vomits and a fever appears. Convulsions and drowsiness may occur, unless the foregoing symptoms are relieved, leading to coma and death.

(b.) Convulsive Variety.—There are no forerunning signs. Instead, convulsions occur, with or without loss of consciousness.

These convulsions may consist of a single attack or a number of attacks, at intervals of a few minutes or several hours. The convulsions resemble epilepsy. The temperature is apt to be high, from 103° to 106° Fahrenheit.

Coma, followed by death, is the frequent ending of this variety of uremia; but the patient may fall into a deep sleep and gradually recover.

(c.) Cerebral Variety or Uremic Coma.—This variety is slow in developing. There is a drowsy feeling, associated with headache and a cross temper. In a short time there are nausea, vomiting and fever, the temperature often going up as high as 107° Fahrenheit. The patient may fall into a coma. The coma is always accompanied by a rise of temperature and stertor. "The stertor is peculiar, it is not the 'snoring' of apoplexy, but a sharp hissing sound, produced by the rush of expired air against the teeth or hard palate."—(Loomis.)

This variety usually terminates fatally. Gradual recovery is rare.

Outcome.—Acute uremia is a very serious condition. The attack may end favorably, but recurrences are common, and the disease finally terminates in death.

TREATMENT.—*During the Attack.* Give a drop of croton oil, diluted by glycerin or sweet oil; or place it on a piece of sugar and place that on the tongue.

Cause free sweating by using the hot pack, vapor bath or hot air bath. (See chapter on Home Nursing.) Poultices over the loins are good. Normal salt solution by rectal injection gives good results. (See chapter on Home Nursing.)

During the Interval. Keep patient in bed and give an enema of magnesium sulphate (one ounce) and caffein citrate (three grains) every three hours. When the secretions have started, give the following powder every two hours for twenty-four hours:

Calomel, one-half grain.
Sodium bicarbonate, two grains.
Powdered ipecac, one-sixth grain.
Make up into powder.

Follow the last dose with some laxative water. It is assumed that a physician will be summoned upon the first appearance of any of the marked symptoms mentioned in the foregoing description of diseases of the kidneys.

Movable Kidney (*Floating Kidney*).—This is a condition of the kidney either dating from birth or acquired in which the tissue and the vessels connected with the kidney are elongated and loosened, thus causing kidney to move in certain directions, like a movable tumor in the abdomen.

Causes.—Some of the causative factors of this disease are the relaxation of the abdominal muscles, from pregnancy or other conditions. The wearing of corsets or girdles that cramp the waist are responsible in many cases for a floating kidney, as well as for other pelvic conditions. Violence, pressure from tumors and rapid emaciation are other causes.

Symptoms.—In the majority of cases, the patient experiences a heavy, dragging pain in the abdomen, made worse by standing or walking, and relieved somewhat when lying down. Disorders of the stomach and intestines, mental worry and hysteria often accompany this condition.

The tendency of the floating kidney is to change its place, and it may be found in the abdomen far from its normal position.

To make a positive diagnosis, a physical examination by a doctor is necessary in every case.

This condition is truly chronic in character, but rarely if ever ends fatally.

TREATMENT.—Do everything to improve the general health of the individual. Give nourishing food, prescribe proper exercise; in other words, follow the laws of good hygiene to the letter.

In many cases the symptoms are relieved by lying on the back. An abdominal supporter that will keep the kidney in place, is strongly advised. When an attack occurs, put the patient in bed, and for the pain a hot fomentation (see Appendix) over the back will prove beneficial. If the attacks occur frequently, a surgical operation, fixing the organ by suturing it in place, may be the best plan to follow. When successful the relief is permanent.

Cystitis (*Catarrh of the Bladder*).—

CAUSES: *Acute Cystitis.*—Some of the causes of the acute variety of this disease are long continued: Partial retention of urine in the bladder, foreign bodies in the bladder, certain kidney affections, inflammation of the urethra, injury or infectious fevers and, especially, diphtheria.

Chronic Cystitis.—This variety may follow the acute form, or may be caused by chronic Bright's Disease, gout, calculi or by the retention of urine, caused by an enlarged prostate or by urethral strictures.

SYMPTOMS: *Acute Cystitis.*—The beginning of

this variety is sudden and is characterized by rigors, slight elevation in temperature, loss of appetite, sleeplessness, a feeling of depression and frequent urination, the urine being passed drop by drop and followed by bladder spasm. There is a dull pain over the bladder and in the groin. The urine is cloudy and has a strong ammoniacal odor.

Chronic Cystitis.—This form progresses slowly and is manifested by a dull pain and frequent, scanty urination. The urine is turbid and contains pus. When allowed to stand, it deposits a thick, glairy sediment.

If an ulceration of the inner membrane of the bladder is present, there will be severe pains localized over the bladder, blood in the urine and loss of weight and strength.

Although the passage of urine is small in amount, if the patient is catheterized, several ounces of ammoniacal, cloudy urine will be drawn off.

Together with these symptoms, those of the underlying condition will be present.

OUTLOOK.—The outlook for acute cases, properly treated, is favorable. The result depends largely upon the nature of the cause.

The chronic variety tends to persist indefinitely and under certain conditions is incurable.

TREATMENT: *Acute Cystitis.*—Put the patient in bed, on a liquid diet, milk being the best. Eliminate highly seasoned articles of food. Warm applications should be placed over the bladder. Large quantities of mineral waters should be taken.

The bowels should be kept freely opened by taking salts.

Chronic Cystitis.—The diet should be milk and the patient should drink freely of alkaline mineral waters. The bladder should be emptied several times a day in order to prevent accumulation and decomposition of the urine. The underlying cause should be treated by a physician.

All cases of cystitis demand the care of a physician as soon as he can be found.

CHAPTER XII

INFECTIOUS AND CONTAGIOUS DISEASES

When the temperature of the body is above normal (98.2° Fahrenheit) the condition is known as Fever. The extent of the fever can be accurately determined only by a clinical thermometer. For the methods of using a thermometer, you are referred to the chapter on Home Nursing.

Degrees of Fever.

When	temperature	is from	99° to 100° F.	condition	is termed	Feverishness.
"	"	"	100° to 101° F.	"	"	Slight Fever.
"	"	"	101° to 103° F.	"	"	Moderate Fever.
"	"	"	103° to 105° F.	"	"	High Fever.
"	"	"	105° to 106° F.	"	"	Intense Fever.
"	"	"	106° F. or over	"	"	Hyperpyrexia.

The decline of the fever may be gradual or sudden. When the fever ends by a sudden drop, the condition is known as *crisis*. When the fever ends gradually, it is known as *lysis*. In most fevers the highest temperature is reached during the evening, usually about 6 P. M., and the lowest temperature in the morning, usually about 6 A. M.

There are three types of fever, namely, continued, remittent and intermittent.

In continued fever, the daily variation is usually from one to one and a half degrees.

In the remittent type, the daily variation is greater, but the lowest daily temperature never reaches the normal point.

In the intermittent type of fever, there are great variations in the temperature, but the lowest daily temperature drops to normal or below.

General Treatment of All Fevers.—When a patient has an appreciable fever, he should be put to bed in a room that is warm but not hot, and where there is good ventilation and quiet.

The feeding should be entirely liquid in character and composed of such foods as milk, beef tea and animal broth. Food should be given in small amounts at frequent but regular intervals. No solid foods should be administered.

The bowels should be kept freely open and sweating should be induced.

For the bowels, give calomel in doses of either a tenth or a quarter of a grain every fifteen minutes until from a grain to three grains have been given; follow this by sulphate of magnesia (Epsom salts), sodium phosphate or one of the various laxative waters.

To induce sweating, hot lemonade, wrapping blankets, etc., should be tried. No drugs should be given to induce sweating, unless recommended by a physician.

To reduce the temperature, the cold pack, cold bath and sponging should be used. See the chapter on Home Nursing for the methods of giving these things.

Besides these points, very little can be done but to call a physician. All fevers are serious ailments and unskilled persons should not attempt to treat them.

In discussing the different fevers, only a bare outline of the treatment will be given. Follow the points under the heading, "General Treatment of All Fevers."

The principal symptoms will be described in order to give some idea of the nature of the disease.

Eruptive Fevers.—Certain fevers are attended by skin eruptions, and the date of their appearance is of vital importance in the diagnosis.

The eruption of German measles appears on the first or second day of illness.

The eruption of measles appears on the third or fourth day.

The eruption of scarlet fever appears on the first or second day.

The eruption of smallpox appears on the third or fourth day.

The eruption of typhoid fever appears on the seventh or ninth day.

The eruption of chicken-pox appears on the first day.

IMMUNITY.—When a person has once had one of the infectious fevers, he is usually immune to a second attack. Such fevers are German measles, chicken-pox, mumps, scarlet fever, typhus, yellow fever, etc.

Typhoid, measles and small-pox sometimes occur a second time.

Simple Continued Fever.—This condition is most common in children. It may be caused by a disordered stomach, mental or physical fatigue, excitement, emotion or exposure to high degrees of heat or cold.

SYMPTOMS.—The beginning is very sudden and may be ushered in with nausea, vomiting, convulsions or a chill. Great weariness and languor accompany these signs. The temperature may run as high as 102° or 103° Fahrenheit, and is accompanied by headache, dry skin, thirst, coated tongue and constipation. Sores are often observed on the lips. The duration is from a few hours to six or eight days. Convalescence is rapid.

Influenza (*Grip, La Grippe*).—Grip will be recognized by the following prominent signs: The sudden onset, chills, followed by fever, temperature reaching 101° to 103° Fahrenheit, severe shooting pains in eyes and forehead, also pains in the joints and muscles, chilliness down the spine, sore throat, hoarseness, deafness, watery eyes, sneezing and a dry cough. Very often there will be pains in the abdomen, nausea, vomiting and diarrhœa.

In mild cases, the fever ends by crisis on the fourth or fifth day. Unless complications occur the convalescence is rapid.

Some of the complications of grip are very grave. Among them may be mentioned pneumonia, cerebro-spinal meningitis, and diseases of the kidneys and heart.

TREATMENT.—Follow the general treatment of all fevers. In grip all the excretions should be disinfected. In the beginning of an attack a hot foot-bath or a hot tub-bath are beneficial.

For the relief of the bronchial symptoms half an ounce of the compound tincture of benzoin in a quart of boiling water, the vapor to be inhaled through the mouth, is beneficial.

Typhoid Fever (*Enteric Fever*).—Before the germ causing typhoid fever was discovered, the disease was called by several names, according to the severity of the attack and the locality in which it occurred. Even to-day, in certain localities, these names still persist. As for example: In mild cases of typhoid the names, gastric fever, slow fever, nervous fever, etc., are applied. In the elevated parts of the Western United States it was and is termed "mountain fever."

The lack of medical knowledge which prevails in places far from medical aid, has led to neglect, and as a result, has caused thousands of new cases and many unnecessary deaths.

Typhoid fever is communicable and is caused by a germ that attacks the intestines chiefly, but which also enters the blood and other parts of the body.

It is most frequent from July to December and between the ages of fifteen and thirty. No age, however, is exempt.

METHODS OF COMMUNICATING TYPHOID FEVER: The germ is always the immediate cause; it reaches the body in various ways.

Water, contaminated through bad drainage, is probably the chief cause of typhoid. Therefore if there is any suspicion that the drinking water is not pure, it should be boiled.

Flies are carriers of typhoid. They alight on the patient or the excreta of a patient and then fly to articles of food. People eating this food are liable to an attack of the disease.

Milk very often, like water, causes typhoid. The milk is put in dirty bottles or cans, is diluted with contaminated water, or is handled by people who have been in contact with patients suffering from typhoid, and so the milk receives the typhoid germ.

Oysters that have grown or been laid in water near the outlet of a sewer, unless they are thoroughly cooked, are liable to convey the disease.

The typhoid germs are always carried into the body with the food and almost never through the lungs. Typhoid germs escape from patients sick with the disease, mainly from the stools and urine; sometimes from the sweat, saliva and vomited matter.

Ice does not kill the typhoid germs. The germ may be in ice for months, and when the ice melts and is consumed by an individual, may cause typhoid fever.

The only way to destroy the germ is by intense heat, as boiling, etc.

Symptoms.—The symptoms of typhoid fever vary in different cases. In this description a typical case will be outlined.

Only the forerunning symptoms are vitally important in order that the disease may be recognized in time.

In no other disease is rest in bed more imperative.

During the first week the onset is gradual. The patient usually cannot tell the day when he first felt sick. The fever mounts a little higher each day. The temperature is at the highest point from the end of the first to the beginning of the third week, being about the same each evening and two degrees lower in the morning. During the third week the fever gradually subsides and convalescence begins, usually after a month's sickness.

The patient is tired, feels lazy, has headaches, backaches, loss of appetite, the muscles feel sore, there are pains in the abdomen, nose-bleed, diarrhœa, coated tongue, flushed face, occasionally vomiting—these or some of these are the signs of typhoid during the first week.

At the end of about ten days pink-red spots, about the size of a pinhead, appear on the abdomen. They number from two to about fifteen, and when pressed disappear, to return when the pressure is withdrawn. These are called "rose spots."

During the second week delirium very often is present. The patient is stupid. The tongue assumes a brownish color and cracks, and the teeth become covered with a brownish material, called sordes.

Diarrhœa is usually present and the stools are of a pea-soup color.

During the third week the general condition begins to improve. The tongue clears and the bowels move less often.

In severe cases the patient becomes weaker. He lies in a stupor and has a muttering delirium, twitching of the fingers and picking at the bedclothes. A patient in delirium must be carefully watched, as he may get out of bed and injure himself.

During the fourth week the temperature falls to normal in the morning, the pulse gets better, the diarrhœa stops and natural sleep returns.

There are many variations from the above description, and numerous complications, which cannot be discussed here.

Treatment.—There is perhaps no disease in which the services of a physician are more necessary than in typhoid fever, on account of its prolonged course and the number of complications which may occur during its existence.

Put the patient to bed, in the horizontal position, at the first suspicion of typhoid. This is to avoid the dangers of bleeding and perforation of the bowels resulting from the ulceration of the structures.

Always use the bed-pan except in case of bleeding from the bowels, in which case use cloths for the discharges instead. It is essential at such a time for the patient to be kept absolutely quiet.

The diet should be liquid. Milk, diluted with water; albumen water, flavored with a few drops of lemon juice, or lactone milk (artificial buttermilk) may be given.

Extreme precautions must be exercised by attendants to escape contracting the disease and to prevent its communication to others. The bed-pan with the stools must be put in 5 per cent. carbolic acid solution and remain in it one hour before being emptied.

The urine should be mixed with an equal part of the same solution and allowed to stand an hour.

Soak all clothing and linen that has been in contact with the patient in carbolic acid solution for two hours. The expectoration must be on old cloths that can be burned.

Any one touching the patient should wash his hands afterward and soak them for a few minutes in a mild antiseptic solution. (See Appendix.)

Cerebro-Spinal Meningitis, Cerebro-Spinal Fever (*Spotted Fever*).—In order to recognize this disease the following points should be kept in mind. The onset is marked by chill, severe headache, persistent nausea, vomiting and fainting. The muscles of the neck and back become rigid and cause an arching. This arching of the head and back is very characteristic. Great restlessness is present and the patient becomes emaciated.

This is a most dangerous disease.

Treatment.—Put the patient to bed away from the others in the house. The bedding, excreta and clothing should be disinfected, as in typhoid fever.

The diet should be composed of milk, eggs, broths, etc., at regular hours.

To the spine and head, ice-bags or cold compresses should be applied.

During convalescence tonics should be given.

Malaria (*Chills and Fevers, Ague*).—Malaria is caused by a plasmodium which enters the body by means of the bites of a certain kind of mosquito.

The principal forms of malaria are intermittent fever, remittent fever and pernicious malaria.

Symptoms.—There is a cold, a hot and a sweating stage. The cold stage is ushered in with a feeling of weariness, headache and nausea. Then the chill begins. It lasts from half an hour to an hour and makes the teeth chatter and the whole body shake.

The skin assumes a pale color and is cold and rough. The features are pinched. The thirst is great and the temperature runs from 102° to 104° Fahrenheit.

Then the hot stage begins. The shivering ceases, the skin becomes hot and flushed and the temperature rises to about 106° Fahrenheit. The patient becomes restless. Severe headache, backache, nausea and thirst are also present. This stage lasts from one to ten hours.

Then the sweating stage begins, the perspiration appearing first on the forehead and slowly extending over the entire body.

All the symptoms abate and the sweating becomes free. This period lasts from one to four hours, after which the patient falls off into a refreshing sleep.

In the remittent or bilious type, the cold stage is moderate and does not return with each attack, and the hot stage is very severe. There are painful headaches and irritability of the stomach. The sweating stage is frequently wanting.

In the pernicious type of malaria, the fever is either remittent or intermittent in character, and there is a congestion of the internal organs. It is rarely seen in the temperate regions, but often occurs in the tropics or sub-tropics.

It may either follow an attack of chills and fever or come on very suddenly.

After the chill, when the hot stage appears, the patient falls into a deep stupor or comatose state, with flushed face, noisy breathing and high fever. Wild delirium or convulsions may be present.

Tho attack may last from six hours to a day, after which the patient may recover and then have another attack, or he may die in the first one.

This is a very grave type of malaria.

Treatment.—*During the Attack.* Give hot drinks and apply hot-water bottles and blankets during the chill. During the hot stage cold sponging of the entire body is beneficial, together with vigorous rubbing.

General Treatment.—Quinine, administered in the proper form and manner, is the one drug to be used in cases of malaria. It can do little or no harm, unless used in large doses for a long time. It is the best policy to buy the best quinine that can be had. Do not take it in pill or tablet form, as these sometimes pass through the bowels undissolved.

Quinine should be taken dissolved in water, or, more agreeably, in starch wafers or gelatin capsules.

As there are types of the chills and fever in

which the attacks occur at stated times, which the patient soon learns to anticipate, the quinine should be given in time to be of some value.

If the attack is due at seven o'clock the drug should be taken five hours earlier. Quinine taken within two hours of the attack is of little or no value. A dose of ten grains of quinine taken three times a day for the first three days, then a dose of five grains three times a day for two weeks, and finally two grains three times daily for the rest of the month of treatment will, in most cases, complete a cure.

If constipation is present, give with the first dose of quinine one-quarter of a grain of calomel every fifteen minutes until two grains have been consumed. This should be followed by a dose of salts.

If a person is going from a healthy section into a malarial district, he should begin taking quinine daily two weeks before reaching his destination, and continue taking it while there.

Erysipelas.—Erysipelas is an acute, specific, infectious disease caused by germs, which gain entrance to the system through some wound or abrasion in the skin or mucous membranes.

It attacks people of all ages, and occurs most frequently in the spring.

The disease usually lasts from three to seven days.

Symptoms.—All the symptoms of fever are present. A patch of red appears on the nose, cheeks, eye or nostril and spreads over the face. It takes on a shining, crimson or violet-hued tinge and has sharply defined edges.

There may be more or less pain, burning or itching and a feeling of tightness present. When it occurs on the face, the features become more or less distorted.

The eruption subsides after four or six days, followed by a moderate peeling of the skin, and the fever abates gradually.

Relapses are not uncommon, but are not so severe as the original attack.

Old people, new-born children and alcoholic subjects are apt to suffer severely and even to die from erysipelas.

Cancer of the skin, chronic skin diseases and old ulcers sometimes follow attacks of erysipelas.

Treatment.—As a rule, erysipelas will run its course and disappear without treatment. Isolate the patient in a room with good ventilation and sunlight. Dressings and other objects coming in contact with the patient must be burned or disinfected.

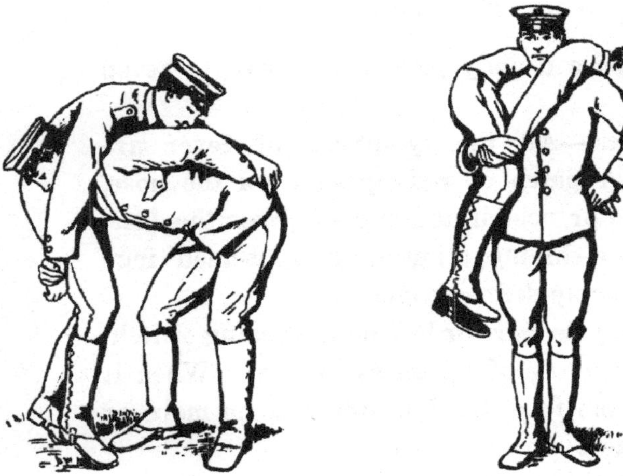

METHOD OF LIFTING AND CARRYING AN INJURED PERSON ACROSS THE SHOULDERS

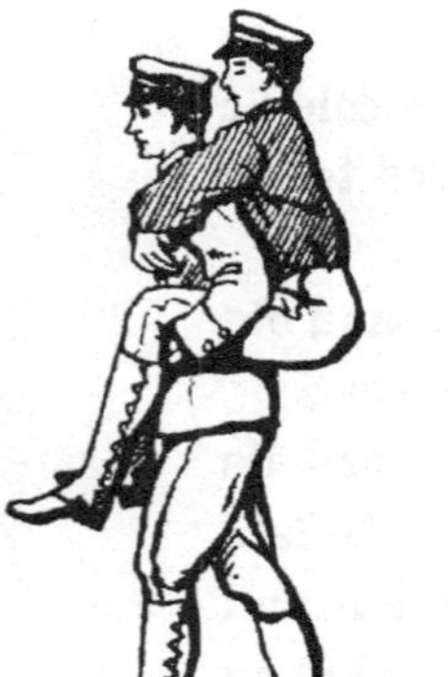

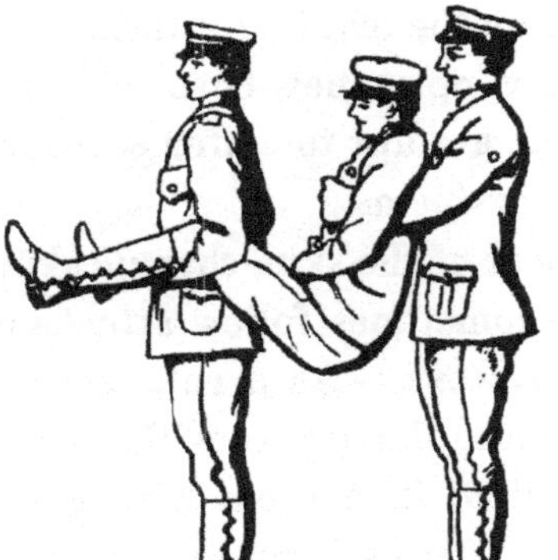

CARRYING AN INJURED PERSON ON THE BACK
METHOD OF CARRYING A PATIENT WHEN THERE ARE TWO ASSISTANTS

A liquid diet of milk, beef tea, broths, etc., is advised. Cloths wet with cold water should be kept over the inflamed area.

For the fever, sponge the body with cold water and alcohol.

The patient must be quarantined until all peeling stops, usually for two weeks.

To be on the safe side and to avoid complications call a physician.

Tetanus (*Lockjaw*).--Lockjaw is caused by a germ, which usually gains access to the body through an abrasion. It frequently follows wounds caused by powder, gunshot, rusty nails, etc., or dirt in wounds from stable refuse.

SYMPTOMS.—The onset is sudden with stiffness of the jaws, neck and tongue and difficulty in swallowing. The stiffness passes down the back muscles to the legs, which are held in a firm spasm. Gradually other spasms develop, involving the muscles of the jaw, causing lockjaw, the face muscles (causing the "sardonic grin") and the neck and trunk muscles.

There is little or no fever, as a rule, but in extreme cases resulting fatally, the temperature runs as high as 108° to 110° Fahrenheit.

The mind remains clear, but any shock, noise or irritation will develop a spasm.

Treatment.—Place the patient at rest in bed in a quiet, darkened room.

The wound will have to be opened and cleaned antiseptically and the tetanus antitoxin administered, as well as stimulation given; therefore a doctor should be sought with all possible haste. Gunshot wounds should be treated in such a manner as to prevent lockjaw.

Yellow Fever (*Yellow Jack, Black Vomit*).—Yellow fever is an acute infectious disease characterized by violent fever, yellow skin and black or "coffee-ground" vomit.

Cause.—The disease is caused by a specific germ carried and communicated to man by a species of mosquito, the *Stegomyia fasciata*.

One attack, as a rule, makes the patient immune to other attacks.

It is most prevalent in tropical countries, but periodic epidemics may occur in other regions.

It is most common during the months of June, July, August and September.

No race, age or sex is exempt from this disease.

Symptoms.—The incubation period is from twenty-four hours to six days.

The *First Stage* is the stage of fever. The disease begins with a tired feeling, headache, loss of appetite and chill. Soon after, the fever begins going up to 104°-106° Fahrenheit; pains are present in the head, limbs and back.

The attack usually begins at night. The patient is nervous and extremely prostrated.

Constipation is the rule. A peculiar and characteristic odor is given off by the patient.

This stage lasts from thirty-six hours to three or four days. During the latter part of this stage the body becomes slightly yellow. If the attack is severe, delirium may be present.

The *Second Stage* is that in which the fever drops to 100° or 99° Fahrenheit. All the symptoms abate and the disease may end by crisis; but, as a rule, after an interval lasting from a few hours to one or four days it passes into the third stage.

The *Third Stage* is that of the secondary fever. All the symptoms return in an exaggerated form. The patient becomes very yellow and then gradually assumes a mahogany color.

A black vomit, bleeding from the mucous membranes, coldness of the surface of the body and irregular breathing may occur.

Death results from exhaustion. The mind remains clear to the end.

Even after the appearance of the black vomit recovery may occur.

Treatment.—Should a person go to a section

where yellow fever is prevalent, or should he live in such a section, the disease may be prevented by screening all living apartments and having a mosquito-proof netting about each bed. There is no danger in the daytime, as the mosquitoes appear only in the hours between sundown and sunrise. When suspicious that a person has yellow fever, he should be put to bed and kept absolutely quiet. There is no danger of "catching" yellow fever from the sick. It must come through the mosquito's bite.

Because of the irritability of the stomach only the mildest of food should be given.

Laxatives, such as castor oil, calomel or citrate of magnesia, may be given.

The stomach irritation may be relieved by cracked ice, milk and lime water or by applying a mustard plaster over the abdomen.

Scarlet Fever.—Scarlet fever is an acute, self-limited, contagious, infectious disease, characterized by a rash and high fever.

SYMPTOMS.—The developing period is from a few hours to a week. The onset is sudden. It is marked by a chill, vomiting or convulsions, followed by sore throat and high fever (105° Fahrenheit).

At the end of a day, a *bright scarlet rash* appears on the neck and chest, which extends over the entire body in a few hours. As soon as the rash is complete, the skin begins to peel. This desquamation or peeling occupies from two to six weeks.

With the rash, the throat-symptoms become prominent. It is difficult to swallow, pain and tenderness are felt in the throat and jaws, the glands of the neck and throat are swollen and the tonsils are inflamed.

At first, the tongue is furred, but later the "strawberry tongue," so called from its reddened appearance, is in evidence. Delirium may be present. The bowels are usually constipated, but a diarrhœa may occur in some cases.

The fever gradually begins to decline on the fourth or fifth day. Convalescence is slow.

Treatment.—Isolate the patient. Put him in bed and insist upon absolute quiet. All the sick-room articles should be carefully disinfected. (Home Nursing.) Playthings, books, etc., should be burned. The bed linen should be soaked in a 5 per cent. carbolic acid solution for a half-hour and then boiled. All cooking utensils should be treated in the same manner.

To reduce the high fever, the cold bath, pack or cool sponging should be tried. (See chapter on

Home Nursing.) Apply an ice-bag to the head.

To keep the bowels open, give one-tenth-grain doses of calomel every half hour for ten doses.

With the appearance of the eruption, the body should be anointed with cold cream or cocoa butter.

Peroxide of hydrogen, diluted by equal parts of water, may be used as a wash and gargle to make the mouth and throat antiseptic.

The complications of scarlet fever are many. To prevent them and to have the proper medical treatment, consult a physician. The convalescing period requires close attention.

Measles.—Measles is an acute, infectious, contagious disease, characterized by catarrhal symptoms, involving the lining membrane of the nose, throat and lungs, fever, and a red mottled rash.

SYMPTOMS.—The incubation period is from ten to fourteen days. The disease begins with a chill or chilliness; fever (101°-102° Fahrenheit), soreness of the muscles, headache and a catarrh of the nose and throat.

Light hurts the eyes, causing them to water. Sneezing and coughing occur.

On the second day the fever falls, and rises again on the fourth day, when the eruption, arranged in crescentic groups, appears on the face. From the face it soon spreads over the entire body. The rash itches and burns. About the ninth day it begins to fade and disappear entirely. A branlike desquamation or peeling takes place. All the symptoms gradually lessen.

OUTCOME.—Nearly all cases that have no complications recover. Lung complications are always serious.

TREATMENT.—Isolate the patient. Put him in bed and protect from drafts. Keep the bowels regular by means of some gentle laxative.

The diet should be of a semi-solid nature. Mild cases require no medicines.

When the temperature becomes too high, give the patient a cold sponge bath.

For the itching, rub on the body cold cream, cocoa butter or similar oily substances.

Camphorated oil, rubbed on the chest and neck, lessens the catarrhal symptoms.

During the convalescence, tonics are advised.

German Measles, French Measles, False Measles (*Rubella*).—An acute, self-limited, contagious disease, characterized by mild fever, suffused eyes, cough, sore throat, enlargement of the glands of the neck and a rose-colored eruption, in patches of irregular size and shape, appearing on the first day.

Many so-called second attacks of measles and scarlet fever are attacks of rubella.—(Tyson.)

SYMPTOMS.—The disease begins suddenly with a mild fever, suffused eyes, but little or no signs of "cold in the head," sore throat, enlargement of the glands of the neck, and a rose-colored eruption, which may appear at any time from the first to the fourth day. Recovery is the rule.

There is no special treatment; the treatment indicated under measles, is applicable to this disease.

Small Pox.—Small-pox is an acute, epidemic and contagious disease, characterized by fever and an eruption.

SYMPTOMS.—The developing period is from ten to sixteen days. The onset is sudden, with a chill, vomiting and excruciating pains in the back and limbs. Within a short time the temperature rises to 103°-104° Fahrenheit.

The face is red. Severe headache, sleeplessness and delirium are often present. The prostration is great.

On the third day the eruption appears on the forehead and lips. This looks like coarse, red spots. Within twenty-four hours the lesions have a shotlike hardness. All other symptoms abate when the eruption appears.

The eruption changes, until on the tenth or eleventh day it begins to dry up, and is converted into scabs or crusts by the end of two weeks.

The features are unrecognizable because of the edema of the skin between lesions.

The scabs or crusts emit a characteristic, offensive odor, and fall off from the seventh day to three weeks, leaving a red, glistening depression or pit. This pit changes into white scar tissue. The secondary fever lasts about three or four days and in favorable cases ends by a gradual decline.

During convalescence, boils, abscesses, eye-disease, ear-trouble and joint-disease are liable to develop.

Treatment.—As soon as you become suspicious of the presence of small-pox, call a doctor.

While waiting for him to come, isolate the patient, put him to bed in a darkened room and give a fluid diet.

All members of the family should speedily be vaccinated. As a rule, all children are vaccinated when young. In the cities, vaccination is required on entering school.

If small-pox is reported in the neighborhood, it is the safest plan to be vaccinated, even though this has been done three or five or seven years before.

Chicken-Pox.—Chicken-pox is a mild, contagious affection, characterized by a moderate fever and an eruption. Children are the ones usually attacked.

SYMPTOMS.—The developing period averages about two weeks. The disease begins with a moderate fever, thirst, loss of appetite and constipation.

The eruption begins as red spots, which rapidly change into clear blisters.

The itching is intense. The rash is most abundant on the trunk.

The blisters dry rapidly and drop or peel off within a week, sometimes leaving pits, if they have been scratched and infected.

Chicken-pox nearly always terminates favorably. Unless complications arise, treatment is unnecessary except to relieve aggravated symptoms.

Mumps.—Mumps is an acute, specific, infectious inflammation of one or both of the glands lying at the angle of the jaw and extending up to the ear (parotid glands), and of other salivary glands.

CAUSES.—It is caused by a specific germ, not yet isolated. It usually occurs in epidemics. The most common ages for it are from five years to puberty; males are more often attacked than females.

SYMPTOMS.—The period of development is from two to three weeks. It begins rather suddenly. The patient feels worn out and languid, and has a chill, which is followed by a fever (101°-103° Fahrenheit), headache, dry skin, and in a day or two stiffness at the angles of the jaw. Then the glands swell and become painful, general edema is present on the affected side, and at times the skin is reddened. Deafness may occur.

The swelling goes down in about a week's time. The health is then restored, or, what is more common, the glands on the opposite side become involved, somewhat postponing recovery.

In severe cases, glands in other parts of the body may become attacked.

TREATMENT.—It is necessary to isolate the patient, insure rest and give a liquid diet.

Locally, hot fomentations are of considerable value in relieving the distress. (See chapter on Home Nursing.)

If the condition becomes severe and other glands swell, a physician should be consulted.

Diphtheria (*Putrid Sore Throat*).—Diphtheria is an acute, specific, constitutional disease, epidemic and contagious, beginning with an affection of the throat; characterized by a local exudation and enlargement of the glands, and fever.

CAUSES.—It is caused by a specific germ.

SYMPTOMS.—The symptoms vary in severity in different cases, and are often disproportionate to the gravity of the attack.

The onset may be mild or severe. In mild cases there are rigors, followed by moderate fever, headache, languor, loss of appetite, stiffness of neck and slight soreness of the throat.

In severe attacks the onset is sudden, with chilliness, followed by a high fever (103°-105° Fahrenheit), and pain in the ear, aching limbs, loss of strength, swelling of neck and painful swallowing. Prostration and weariness are very marked.

The local symptoms are associated with the throat. The throat is seen to be red, swollen and spotted.

A false membrane forms, which can be removed, leaving a bleeding surface. A new, dirty white membrane promptly forms.

In severe cases, ulceration and sloughing may be observed.

The breath has an offensive odor. The glands of the neck are enlarged and tender.

An offensive discharge from the nose is present, with attacks of nose-bleed.

Hoarseness or loss of the voice, croupy cough, shortness of breath and noisy breathing are commonly observed.

The disease lasts from two to fourteen days. Complications may prolong its course. Relapses are not uncommon.

TREATMENT.—To make a positive diagnosis, a laboratory examination of the exudation from the throat must be made. If found to be diphtheretic, the antitoxin is advised in all cases. Therefore, if diphtheria is suspected, lose no time in calling a doctor.

The patient should be isolated and all means taken to prevent the spread of the disease. Rest in bed is essential.

Employ a diet composed of milk, eggs, broths, oysters, etc., and feed every two hours.

If swallowing is painful or difficult, feed the patient by the rectum. (See chapter on Home Nursing.)

The atmosphere of the room should be rendered warm and moist.

Direct inhalations of hot steam are beneficial. Sponges soaked in hot water and applied to the throat afford relief.

Keep the bowels regular by the use of laxatives.

In diphtheria the same sick-room precautions must be observed as in scarlet fever.

Whooping Cough.—Whooping cough is an infectious disease characterized by fits of coughing, consisting of a number of forcible expirations, during which a long-drawn breath is followed by a whooping or crowing sound.

Causes.—It is a contagious disease, believed to be due to an unknown germ, associated with the sputum.

It is a disease of childhood, although adults may be affected. One attack usually renders the patient immune to subsequent attacks.

Symptoms.—Whooping cough may be divided into three stages: catarrhal, spasmodic and terminal.

The catarrhal stage, lasting two weeks, begins as an ordinary cold with a loose cough.

The spasmodic stage lasts about four weeks, and consists of attacks of from fifteen to twenty short coughs without drawing breath. The face swells, grows red or blue, the eyeballs protrude, the veins become prominent and the patient appears to be suffocating. When at last he draws in a long breath, a whooping sound is caused, giving rise to the name of this disease.

The attacks of coughing may be followed by

vomiting. If the vomiting occurs shortly after food has been taken, the nutrition of the patient will suffer. Profuse nose-bleed is frequent.

During the terminal stage, the attacks happen at longer intervals, are shorter in duration and less in intensity. The catarrhal signs are more marked and the expectoration is freer. The duration of this stage is from one to two weeks. The patient often develops the "cough of habit."

TREATMENT.—The disease is self-limited and there is no specific treatment.

The patient should be isolated together with his personal articles, in order to prevent the spread of the disease. There is no need to put the sick one to bed, but he should be kept in a light, airy room.

On clear days he should be allowed the open air, being careful to protect him from taking cold.

The diet should be nutritious and composed of articles of which the patient is fond.

During convalescence tonics are of great value.

CHAPTER XIII

DISEASES OF CHILDREN

CHILDREN and adults have many diseases in common. These ailments are described in other parts of this book. The following chapter mentions only the diseases which are peculiar to and common in children.

Inflammation of the Breasts in the New-Born Child.—This condition in babies a few days old is not an uncommon occurrence. The breasts of the infant become swollen and tender. The child cries more than the normal baby. A few drops of a milky looking liquid may be excreted from the nipples. In rare cases, the breasts may become infected and abscesses form. Then the swelling increases, the breasts become very red and matter or pus forms. In the simple inflammation, the appetite is not disturbed and no fever is present. But in the case of pus the appetite is impaired and a fever is present. Such cases should be referred to a doctor in order that an incision in the breasts may be made to relieve the trouble.

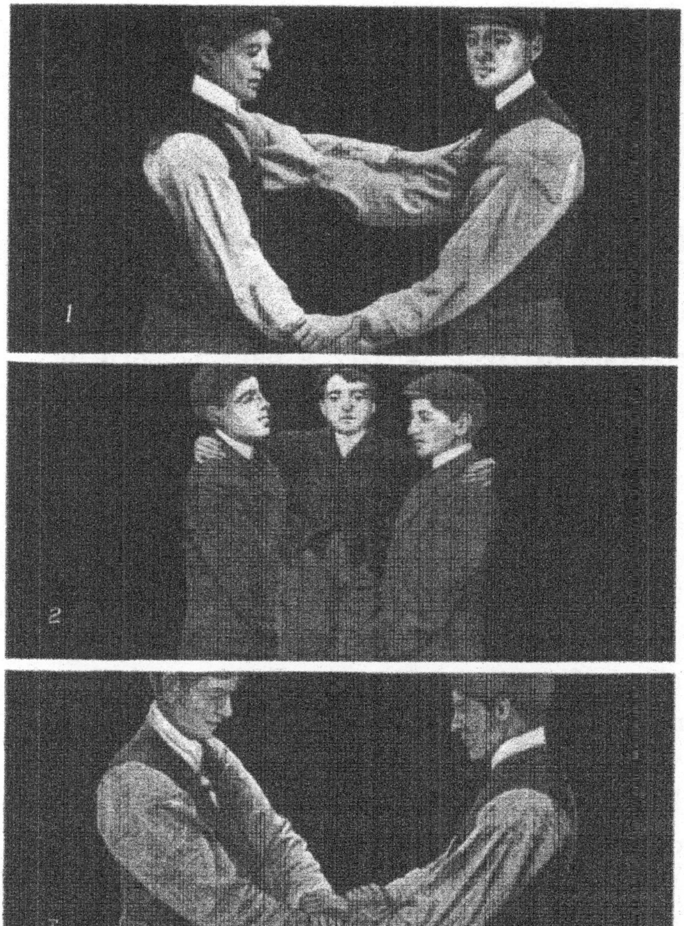

1. TWO-HANDED SEAT AND SHOULDER REST. MAY BE USED FOR UNCONSCIOUS PATIENTS
2. PATIENT IN SUCH A SUPPORT
3. FOUR-HANDED SEAT. PATIENT MUST BE ABLE TO SUPPORT HIMSELF WITH HIS ARMS

As a rule, the simple cases will subside without treatment. It would be better, however, to wash the breasts with warm water and soap, and then put on a dressing made by soaking cloths with a solution of boric acid (one teaspoonful to two glasses of water). A fresh dressing should be applied daily.

Retention of Urine.—After a baby is born, it may pass no urine for twenty-four to thirty-six hours. This should not alarm the parents, especially if the child is a boy. If after twelve hours it has not passed urine, put the baby in a warm bath, and very often this will produce the desired result. After a day, or a day and a half, if the urine has not been voided it will be the safest plan to consult a doctor. A malformation may be present that will need prompt treatment.

If the baby has a severe attack of colic, the urine will be suppressed, but this condition will be relieved by a warm bath.

If the diapers are stained with a reddish or yellowish deposit from the urine it shows that the urine is too concentrated. The passage of such urine is very painful. Give the baby plenty of water and this condition will disappear.

If the natural opening for the passage of urine in a male infant is as small as a pinhole, which may happen, and if this opening is not enlarged, this condition, if it persists as the child grows, may cause trouble. The parts become sore, red and swollen; the passage of urine becomes painful; the irritation may lead to bad habits; bed-wetting is common; various nervous diseases, such as St. Vitus' dance, spasm and general nervousness may result, and a prolapse of the bowel may be caused by the child straining to pass his urine.

The patient should be examined by a doctor if any of the above symptoms are present, as the difficulty can easily be remedied by him.

Bleeding of the Cord and Infection of the Navel. —After the baby has been born and the doctor or attendant has left, bleeding may occur from the navel cord. This may be stopped by tying, as tightly as possible, a soft string, or, what is better, narrow tape about the cord. If the bleeding cannot be controlled, seek medical aid.

If oozing is present after the cord drops off, there is no cause for alarm.

In rare cases the cord will become soft, have a foul odor and drop off, leaving a large sore. "Matter" may be discharged. For this a physician should be consulted, as very serious results may follow, but while waiting for the doctor to come, it should be washed three times a day with a solution of one teaspoonful of boric acid to two glasses of water. Clean the part with cheesecloth or absorbent cotton, then dust with dry boric acid, and cover with clean gauze or cotton.

Marasmus (*Wasting*).—Marasmus is a condition in which there is a wasting of the tissues, caused by defective nutrition. It is observed during the first years of life.

It is caused by feeding infants by the bottle with improper food; by giving undiluted milk, unsuitable patent foods, cereals, vegetables, meat or bread before the baby is two years of age.

Naturally, the baby cannot digest such food and so starves. Lack of cleanliness in the care of bottles and rubber nipples; and artificial food contribute to cause marasmus.

SYMPTOMS.—A rapid and progressive loss of weight is the main symptom. When the baby is several months old it may weigh less than when it was born.

The eyes are sunken and squint. The skin is sallow, wrinkled and hangs in folds. The lips are thin and pale.

The baby looks like a little "old man."

Very often patches of sores are present about the buttocks and on the inner surfaces of the thighs. The tongue is coated and dry.

Colic is frequent and sometimes diarrhœa and vomiting occur. The stools look like curds or lumps covered with a green colored slime.

The appetite is often ravenous.

The baby sucks the thumb or hand until it is raw. It also cries or dozes most of the time.

As a rule, the temperature is below normal.

TREATMENT.—In order to treat this disease successfully, the cause must be discovered. After this has been removed and proper feeding instituted, an improvement will be seen at once. Rubbing sweet oil on the body after a warm bath twice a day will prove beneficial.

Marasmus is a very serious condition, which in many cases ends fatally. The parents should not experiment with the treatment, but call in a doctor.

Rickets.—Rickets is a constitutional disease peculiar to children, and characterized by changes in the bones and defects of nutrition.

It is common in certain types of infants between the ages of six months and three years.

The most important causes are improper food and water, or the absence of a necessary amount of fresh cow's milk.

It is a disease of large cities, where the poor live crowded together under unhygienic conditions.

Breast-fed infants do not usually develop rickets unless nursed more than nine months, or unless the mother becomes pregnant again while nursing. Feeding the baby poor patent baby-foods or condensed milk will sometimes cause rickets. Boiled water given exclusively will cause rickets; always give filtered water.

SYMPTOMS.—The first signs of this disease to be noticed are restlessness, sweating about the head and a disposition to throw off the bed-clothes at night.

At times a slight fever will be present. The baby cries when moved because of soreness of the body.

The abdomen is distended, giving the "pot-bellied" look.

The flesh is soft and flabby, but often there is no loss of weight.

Later, in the course of the disease, after the child walks, it may have bow-legs, a pigeon breast or a lateral curvature of the spine.

Changes in the Bones.—The changes in the bones furnish indications for positive diagnosis.

On the ribs, running from the breast-bone outward and downward, are little beadlike lumps that are easily felt. Because of the feeling, it has been called the rachitic rosary.

There is an enlargement of the bones at the wrist.

The shape of the head is characteristic. It is often large, and either square with a projecting forehead and flat sides and top, or it is long with a flat top.

The fontanelle (soft spot), which in a healthy child should close at from fourteen to eighteen months, remains open until the child is three or four years of age.

The teeth are late in appearing. They are usually small, uneven and decay easily.

OUTCOME.—Rickets in itself is not a fatal disease. But a child with rickets is susceptible to colds, coughs, diarrhœa, difficult breathing, convulsions and other troubles common in children.

The deformities in the bones are permanent. As a rule, the child's growth is stunted, and in women who had rickets in childhood there is present a deformity of the hips, which either makes childbirth very hard or impossible.

TREATMENT.—Keep the babies out of doors as much as possible. Do not permit the child to stand or walk too early. This is accomplished by applying splints which extend below the feet.

A daily warm sponge bath, followed by rubbing the body with sweet oil, is beneficial.

The most important part of the treatment is the feeding, and a doctor should be consulted to arrange a proper diet for the baby.

Scrofula (*Enlarged Glands*).—Situated in the armpit, along the sides of the neck and under the lower jaw are chains of glands, called lymphatic glands, which in the healthy person cannot be felt.

From various causes these glands become enlarged, suppurate and may break down.

If a person has an infection, the lymphatic glands near it will become enlarged and tender. For the same reason, if an abnormal condition arises in the nose or throat, the glands of the neck and jaw will become enlarged. Adenoids, a sore throat, inflammation of the tonsils, sore mouth and tongue, abscess of the ear, eczema of the scalp, germ diseases, as measles, scarlet fever, diphtheria, or decayed or loose teeth, will cause an enlargement of the glands.

Cure the primary cause and the glands will return to their normal state.

But the majority of enlarged glands are caused by the tuberculosis germ. It is common to call tuberculous people scrofulous.

Tuberculosis may exist in any part of the body except the hair, nails and teeth. When the glands of the neck are attacked, they become enlarged, and scrofula (an antiquated term) results.

The glands enlarged from this cause are most often seen in children under ten years of age. Sometimes the germ attacks the healthy glands directly, but, as a rule, the glands have been enlarged from other causes, and while in such a state tuberculosis germs enter.

The tuberculous glands develop slowly. One or two lumps are felt. They are not painful or tender. After a while they enlarge, become tender on pressure, grow painful, soften and form abscesses, which may rupture, forming discharging wounds.

When a gland suddenly enlarges and then vanishes spontaneously, you may rest assured it is not tuberculous. If such glands become tender and form abscesses, this will happen a short time after their appearance. In the tuberculous variety, the abscess forms long after the disease was first discovered.

Tuberculous glands, after persisting for a long time, may disappear spontaneously.

Treatment.—In all cases the cause of the enlarged glands must be discovered. This, of course, necessitates the services of a physician.

If the cause be an abnormal condition of the

throat, nose, mouth or ear, such as adenoids, inflamed tonsils, etc., they should be removed.

It often takes some time to be sure the glands are tuberculous. When the diagnosis is positively made, the most important item in the treatment is the hygiene of the patient. Such patients should live out of doors as much as possible, and eat plain, nourishing food, with an abundance of butter and cream. Cod liver oil, taken before each meal, is a valuable aid in the treatment. Mild exercises should be indulged in, such as bathing, golf, walking, etc. Tennis is too strenuous. Late hours, social excitement and dissipation, and too little sleep, all tend to increase the severity of the disease.

By "right living" a cure or an abatement of the trouble may result in many cases. An operation is, by no means, always necessary. But when the enlarged glands persist, grow in size and number, soften and form abscesses, surgical interference is necessary.

Chorea (*St. Vitus's Dance*).-This is a nervous disorder, usually affecting children between the ages of five and fifteen. No age, however, is immune, and it occasionally attacks pregnant women. Girls suffer from it oftener than boys.

CAUSES.—It may be caused by sudden mental

excitement, intestinal worms, dentition, eye-strain, etc.

Although it is not entirely understood, there exists a close relationship between acute rheumatism and chorea. Anemia or malnutrition are among the exciting causes. A tendency to the disease exists in certain families.

SYMPTOMS.—The onset of chorea is generally gradual. The child becomes nervous, cannot sit still, cries easily, often has night terrors and pains in the legs and stomach-ache.

He makes grimaces or jerks the arm or hand. These symptoms are followed by irregular movements of the muscles of the face, or the eyeballs, of the eyelids and the shoulder, arm and hand. The patient is apt to be misjudged, as being wilful and purposely awkward. Sometimes the nervous movements extend to the lower extremities, interfering greatly with walking. In severe cases, there is inability on the part of the patient to feed himself or hold anything in the hands.

Often the speech is unintelligible, as the tongue constantly moves in an irregular manner.

The movements may be almost continuous, or there may be long periods of quiet. The movements are much worse when the patient is tired.

The muscles are usually still during sleep, although this is not always the case. The mind is somewhat blunted, the temper fretful and irritable, and there is a varying degree of mental weakness in this disease, from a state of deficient memory to temporary insanity in rare cases.

St. Vitus's Dance tends to run a course of from eight to ten weeks, with recovery when the treatment is begun in the early stages.

Relapses are frequent, and the spring is the time when the disease returns.

Accompanying chorea may be a chronic heart disease.

TREATMENT.—The child should be removed from all mental and physical excitement. It is better to keep him away from every one except the nurse. Never punish him because of the grimaces or movements he makes. The surroundings should be absolutely hygienic.

Many cases improve rapidly when confined to a bed in a darkened room.

The diet should be light and the bowels should be kept freely open with salines.

The cause should be removed if possible. All reflex irritation, such as accompanies eye-strain, intestinal parasites, dental disorders, etc., should receive proper attention.

A physician will prescribe the proper drugs for this disease.

Spinal Disease (*Hunchback*).—This disease is technically known as Pott's Disease. It is caused by a softening and destruction of a portion of the bones of the spine, due to tubercular germs. Usually it begins in children between the ages of three and five.

If it goes on without treatment it eventually leads to deformity of the spine, or "hunchback." As the anterior part of the bones softens, the support of the back is impaired at that point and the posterior part of the spine is bowed outward, causing the deformity.

The seat of this disease is generally in the upper two-thirds of the back. A blow or a fall received a long time before the spinal trouble became known may have been the exciting cause, but the tubercular germ is responsible for the condition.

SYMPTOMS.—The progress of this disease is slow. Before any definite signs appear, the child is fretful, lies on the floor, and will not stand or play. It often has a cough or pain in the abdomen.

The important symptoms are pain, stiffness of the back, weakness and deformity.

The pain is not felt, except when the child is jarred. He often cries out in his sleep, owing to unconscious movements. When the spine is pressed, tenderness will usually be found.

Stiffness of the back is a characteristic sign. The child does not bend its back freely, but carries itself stiffly. When it wishes to pick up anything, it does not bend as would a healthy child, but squats down by bending the legs at the knees and hips.

As a rule, this disease is not noticed by the parents, until the deformity is well established. This is unfortunate, as the earlier the physician begins treatment, the better are the results.

The deformity is observed as a knuckle-like projection in some part of the back, and is better seen by bending the back.

If the spine in the upper part of the back and neck is attacked by the tubercular germ, the shoulders are apt to be held high and a chronic stiff neck is usually present.

TREATMENT.—As soon as there is a suspicion of spinal disease, a physician should be consulted, in order to begin treatment. There is nothing to do but to place the child in hygienic surroundings until the doctor comes.

Lateral Curvature.—Lateral curvature is due to a bowing of the spine at one side, giving the latter the appearance of the letter S. It results from causes which tend to pull the spine out of line, and, as in early childhood the tissues are soft, permanent distortion occurs.

A faulty position of the body is very often a cause of this disease. Badly arranged desks at school, the carrying of heavy weights, paralysis of the muscles on one side of the body, or loss of an arm, rickets, etc., may cause this trouble.

As a rule, the deformity does not become apparent until the child grows up (from eight to fifteen years of age).

To make sure of the curvature, mark a straight line along the parts of the spine down the back.

Usually no unpleasant symptoms are present.

TREATMENT.—As this deformity may sometimes be corrected by proper exercise and apparatus, as soon as it is noticed a physician should be informed. Parents should be on the lookout for the presence of this form of spinal trouble.

Hip-Joint Disease.—Hip-joint disease is an inflammation of the hip, usually caused by the tubercular germ.

SYMPTOMS.—The course of the disease is gradual.

The first sign noticed is usually a slight limp and stiffness of the diseased limb in the morning, which passes off after the child plays awhile. Recurrences are common, and each succeeding attack is worse than the previous one. A little later there is pain with the lameness.

The pain, at first, is in the toe, calf of the leg or knee. These pains are often called "growing pains" by the parents. "Growing pains," as a rule, are really rheumatism, a sign sufficient to alarm the intelligent parent.

The child cries out in the night because of the pains. The position in which he holds the affected limb is characteristic of tuberculosis of the hip.

The healthy limb bears the weight of the body, while the affected limb is bent slightly at the thigh, and the toes and leg are turned outward. The crease, naturally present under the buttocks, is less noticeable on the leg of the affected side.

If discovered soon enough, nearly all cases can be cured by rest in bed, splints and apparatus of various kinds.

If neglected, an abscess forms about the joint. This condition takes a long time to cure, causes years of suffering, permanent crippling and lameness, and sometimes loss of the limb, or perhaps death.

CHAPTER XIV

SURGICAL CONDITIONS

This chapter does not pretend to cover all surgical conditions. It simply takes the most usual conditions and those which the layman most easily recognizes, and lays down the general course to be followed in their treatment.

One aim of this chapter is to impress upon the reader the importance of noticing any abnormal growth or deformity he may have, any sudden change in his physical condition, such as an abscess, a hernia, etc., and the further importance of reporting such conditions promptly to a doctor. No one but a trained physician understands what may result from neglect of any of these things. The layman too often waits until pain and disability drive him to a doctor, where he finds that pain and disability are the last symptoms to develop of a serious condition, and that if he had gone to a doctor earlier he might have been cured.

Deformities.—Children are sometimes born

with deformities, such as hare-lip, webbed fingers or toes, cleft palate, birthmarks, club feet and many other similar defects. The parents are the ones on whom the responsibility rests for correcting these deformities. Modern surgery does wonders, and it is during childhood that the best results are obtained. Hence, the supreme duty a parent owes to such an unfortunate child is to see that some good surgeon has a chance to correct Nature's error. The poor have the same opportunity as the rich, at least in cities, for in all the free dispensaries and hospitals the best surgeons work for nothing, so that they may perfect themselves in their art.

Growths and Tumors.—There are many different forms of tumors and growths, none of which need be fully explained in this place: they are for the physician to grapple with. But the layman should know the following points:

1. The gradual or sudden appearance of any swelling or lump anywhere on the body means the presence of some tumor, cyst (a sac filled with fluid) or other growth. These may be harmless in their action on the body (as a wen or a fatty tumor) or they may be very harmful, even affecting life itself. The layman should never trust his own judgment nor that of his friends. Always

consult a competent physician *as soon as such a growth is noticed.*

2. Internal growths cannot be felt by a layman until a late stage of their development is reached. But there are warning symptoms that should send any intelligent persons to a physician. Gradual and continued loss of weight, strength and appetite are the most prominent. A peculiar, yellowish-white, wrinkled look to the skin is noticeable. These symptoms, long before there is any pain, should send a man to his physician.

Hernia (*Rupture*).—The protrusion of any organ from its proper cavity is called a hernia. The protruded parts are generally contained in a bag, formed by the membrane which naturally lined the cavity. The most frequent hernias are in the abdominal cavity.

An abdominal hernia occurs when the abdominal wall weakens, the muscle fibers separate and a part of the contents of the abdomen protrudes. Gradually the rupture enlarges, and more of the contents, usually intestines, escape. They lie in a sac, covered only with the skin and some muscle fibers. These sacs sometimes become very large. Others have such a small opening that the intestines are caught in them and cannot get back. If the pressure is great, the blood supply is cut off.

The hernia is then called strangulated, and unless relieved by an operation will cause decay (or gangrene) of the intestines and death. If such a strangulation occurs, the patient feels a sudden terrible pain, he becomes cold, clammy and weak; his face is pale, sunken and terrified, an operation has to be performed immediately to save his life.

But many people have "ruptures" for years without such a condition occurring. These people wear a truss or support for their rupture. Unless there is some good reason why the patient should not be operated on, a truss is a very poor substitute for an operation. The latter cures; the former only alleviates.

Children, especially boys, often have hernias. Parents should not let them grow up in that condition. They are not only barred from all positions in the army, navy, police and fire departments, but they are continually in danger of the condition of strangulated hernia, with its menace to life, and they suffer pain and inconvenience from the truss. The operation has almost no danger to life, and cures absolutely in the great majority of cases.

Furuncle (*Boil*).—A boil is a local infection of the skin, accompanied by the formation of pus. Some boils extend into the deeper tissue, which becomes necrotic and forms the "core" of the boil.

Boils occur in all parts of the body. If the skin is thin and tender they come to a head easily and rupture spontaneously, discharge their pus or "matter" and get well. But in a thicker, stronger skin they are under greater tension, they spread more, and usually to obtain the best results, they should be opened by a doctor. Never poultice boils, and do not delay to seek medical aid. After the rupture or incision of an abscess, perfect cleanliness is necessary, for if the pus is allowed to run over the skin, other hair follicles will become infected and a series of boils will result.

Carbuncle.—This is a collection of boils, in one place, which involves the deeper tissues and tends to spread in all directions. It is a serious affection, causing great exhaustion and even death. The back of the neck is the most usual place for a carbuncle, although it may appear anywhere. Extensive gangrene (death of the tissues) results in a carbuncle.

Early medical advice is necessary. After the doctor has made the neccessary incisions, wet solutions are kept on the neck, the patient is kept quiet, well fed and carefully nursed. A poor general condition accompanies a carbuncle, and must be treated as energetically as the local trouble itself.

Abscess.—This is a local inflammatory condition which begins deeper than the skin. Pus is formed just as in a boil. A gland which has been inflamed and then "broken down," as it is called, is often the origin of an abscess. Abscesses occur in the appendix, in the liver, brain, glands of the neck, arm and body and in many other places. They are felt as red, hot, painful, throbbing swellings. This does not apply to tubercular abscesses, which form slowly with no redness or pain.

These abscesses must all be treated by a physician. Do not delay, for the period of convalescence is greatly shortened by early treatment.

Appendicitis.—This is an inflammation of the appendix, a small organ attached to the cæcum, or pouchlike beginning, of the large intestine. It lies in the right lower side of the abdominal cavity. The inflammation may be of various kinds and of varying degrees of severity.

Causes.—Indigestible food, constipation, exposure to cold, causing an enteritis (inflammation of the intestines), foreign bodies, such as seeds and concretions of the feces (or fecoliths, as they are termed), all tend to start an appendicitis.

Symptoms.—Pain in the right lower side of the

abdomen usually. At the beginning of an attack, the pain is sometimes referred to the upper abdomen, in the middle, so that the sufferer thinks he has gastric colic. On pressure, there is great tenderness of the abdominal wall, and it is rigid and boardlike on the right side, in comparison to the left side. There is usually constipation, coated tongue, loss of appetite and some fever. The patient lies in bed, huddled up, with the right leg and knee drawn up in bed.

TREATMENT.—When these symptoms are present, a doctor should be called, for at the early stage of this inflammation the best results from operation are obtained. If no doctor can be reached, do as follows:

Put the patient in bed and apply an ice-bag to his right side. Always cover the ice-bag with a thick cloth to prevent freezing the skin. Keep this ice-bag filled steadily, except for a few moments in every hour, when the skin should be allowed to warm up a little. Give the patient a good dose of castor oil or olive oil if it is the first day of illness. Later, give only enemas; keep the bowels well emptied with these enemas. Never give salts or other violent purgatives. Feed the patient on milk only. Keep track of his temperature and pulse, and get a physician as soon as possible.

A person who has had one attack of appendicitis and recovered without an operation is almost sure to have another at some later date. It is best to have it out at the first attack or else to have what is termed an "interval" operation. By this we mean an operation in the interval between attacks. This greatly lessens the operative danger and insures a shorter period in bed.

It is most unwise to delay in any case of appendicitis. The best physicians and surgeons usually advise prompt operation. No one can tell at the beginning of an attack how severe it will be. If neglected the appendix may go on to form an abscess, which will rupture, discharging the matter from it into the abdomen cavity, and a condition of peritonitis will result. This is an inflammation of the lining of the cavity and it is one of the gravest complications of appendicitis. A large percentage of peritonitis cases die.

There is another important fact to be considered. If a case is operated upon in the early stages, before an abscess has formed, the wound is what is called "clean," and may be completely closed up. The time in bed is then about two weeks. If the operation is delayed until after the abscess formation, the wound is dirty and cannot be sewed up entirely. A drain through which the "matter" may escape must be left, and this means four or five weeks in bed before this drain closes up.

There is another form of appendicitis, called the gangrenous form. The onset is very sudden and its outcome is grave. The blood supply becomes shut off by swelling or pressure, and in a few hours, twelve to twenty-four at the most, the appendix is gangrenous and rotting. There is little pain with this form except at first. There is no fever, but there is a great deal of shock. The patient's face shows he is very ill. It is sunken, pale, haggard. The abdomen is rigid on the right side. Immediate operation is the only treatment for this condition.

Hemorrhoids (*Piles*), Fissures and Fistulas of the Rectum.—These are three very common and painful conditions of the rectum and anus.

Hemorrhoids, or "piles," as they are commonly called, are caused by the permanent dilation and protrusion of the veins which surround the rectum. They become engorged with blood, which sometimes clots. These masses interfere with defecation and make it very painful. They sometimes bleed very excessively.

The best preventive of hemorrhoids is to keep from constipation, and if one already has hemorrhoids the best way to prevent pain and increased hemorrhoids is to keep the bowels open and the movements soft. Compound licorice powder is the best cathartic to take in such a case. It makes a free, soft stool which does not irritate the rectum.

People who suffer much from piles should not delay to have them operated on. There is no danger to the patient, the relief is great, and the cure is usually permanent. If an operation cannot be obtained, the piles may be helped by bathing them daily in alum solution or anointing at night with 10 per cent. nutgall ointment. These preparations shrink and harden the piles. This treatment, combined with a daily loose movement, will keep a patient fairly comfortable.

An anal fissure is a crack of the skin of the anus. It is usually caused by some particularly hard constipated movement. These fissures are intensely painful, and owing to the daily movement passing over them they never heal spontaneously. A doctor must be called to treat them. Usually a slight operation is necessary.

A rectal fistula is a passage leading from the rectum to the outside, through which fecal matter is discharged. These occur alongside of the anus or natural opening. Some fistulas are incomplete; that is, they lead from the rectal wall into the surrounding tissue, but do not open externally. They are very painful, they tend to spread and enlarge, and are often tubercular in origin. The pain of fistula is enough to drive any one to a doctor. Operation is the only sure means of cure, and if advised by the physician should be unhesitatingly agreed to by the patient.

Felon (*Whitlow*).—A felon is an inflammation of the tendon sheath, accompanied by the formation of pus. A felon usually occurs on some part of the hand. The pain is intense, and of a throbbing, shooting nature. The finger is swollen, hard and very tender. Matter forms in the sheath, and as it is easier for it to pass up the sheath rather than break through the skin, there is danger of general infection unless surgical aid is sought.

TREATMENT.—*Never poultice a felon.* This is the worst possible treatment for it and many a patient has lost his finger, or at least rendered it stiff and useless, as a result of this treatment. Put on a wet dressing of salt water, or boric acid, as hot as can be borne, and then seek a doctor. The felon must be cut open, to allow the matter to escape, and the sooner this is done the quicker the cure.

Gangrene of a Part.—This is the death of any tissue and there are several causes for it.

1. An injury which crushes the part or cuts off its blood supply.

2. In diabetes, gangrene of the toes or fingers occurs sometimes spontaneously.

3. Carbolic gangrene occurs when any person has continuously used a carbolic solution with which to keep any part moist. For this reason carbolic solutions should not be used without a doctor's order.

Treatment.—Amputation of the gangrenous part is the only thing to be done. Hence, consult a doctor promptly.

CHAPTER XV

THE CARE OF THE INFANT

NOTE.—The writers are indebted, for many valuable points on the care of Infants, to Dr. L. Emmet Holt's books, entitled *Diseases of Children* and *The Care and Feeding of Children*, and to Dr. Edward Ellis's *Diseases of Children*.

Care of the Baby Immediately After Birth.

The Cord.—The physician will have tied the navel cord, applied alcohol to the stump and dressed it with cotton, or, which is preferable, a padding of sterile gauze, with an opening for the stump.

In caring for the baby, the cord should be examined every few hours. If it bleeds, boil some narrow tape or cotton and tie it tightly about the stump. As a rule, the cord drops off about the fifth day, leaving a small raw spot. This should be cleansed by pouring on water which has been previously boiled, and then dusting with dry boric acid. Then apply a gauze pad. Do not worry if the cord should not drop off for a week or ten days.

The Binder.—A binder or belly-band, about four inches in width, and long enough to encircle the body and overlap about three inches, should be worn during the first six months. While the cord remains, it should be turned to the left side of the infant before the binder is applied. The liver is on the right side and any pressure may prove harmful.

After the baby is six months of age, a knitted band may be used for two years.

Anointing the Baby.—After tying and dressing the cord the baby is anointed all over with either warm sweet oil or vaseline. Then wrap it in flannel and place in a warm, dry place. Do not bathe for several hours.

Bathing.—After a few hours the cheesy matter on the body may be washed off. Use warm water and some bland, pure soap. Do not put the baby into a bath-tub until it is from ten to fifteen days old. Keep a new-born baby flat on its back or stomach.

If the baby is strong, sponge it with warm water daily during the first fortnight, but if weak and feeble rub it with warm olive oil.

After ten or fifteen days the baby should be given a daily tub-bath. The water should be 100° Fahrenheit. Use a soft, boiled cloth to wash it with and not a sponge. It is impossible to keep a sponge clean.

First, wash the head and face, soap the body and then put in the tub. Support the head and back and wash off the soap. For the buttocks use a separate cloth. Dry the baby with a soft towel. Do not rub the skin. Avoid any irritation.

If the skin is very delicate, put a bag of cheese-cloth containing a pint of bran into the water for five minutes before the bath, and then squeeze it thoroughly.

Avoid all drafts and chilling. Before bathing the baby, have the room heated to a temperature slightly warmer than normal (70°-75° Fahrenheit).

Wash the eyes with a solution of boric acid—one teaspoonful to a pint of water. If the eyes become red, swollen and discharge matter, send for a physician at once. The majority of cases of blindness are due to ignorance concerning the eyes of the newly born infant.

Prevent chafing by changing soiled diapers and cleansing the child at once. Dust a reliable dusting powder in the folds of the skin, or rub with olive oil or cocoa butter.

If a rash appears on the body, stop all bathing until it is gone, and seek the advice of a physician.

After six months the temperature of the bath may be reduced to 95° Fahrenheit, and after one year and up to three years to 90° Fahrenheit.

Clothing.—The baby's clothes should be loose and hang from the shoulders. Do not overdress the infant. In summer, use the thinnest gauze shirts, and in winter a medium weight of flannel.

In the winter, when the infant goes out of doors, thick warm coats and leggings are better than heavy flannels. If this point is observed, the baby will not be so likely to suffer from "colds."

Temperature of the Nursery.—For the first three months, during the daytime, the temperature of the nursery should be kept at about 68° Fahrenheit. At night-time it should never be below 65° Fahrenheit. Do not open the windows during the first month, unless the child is born during the warm months. After a year, the temperature can be as low as 45° Fahrenheit. The nursery should be aired after the bathing time and before bedtime.

Do not cook, wash or dry clothes in the nursery. The room should be bare of hangings, pictures or upholstery and should be of fair size and sunshiny.

If possible, the heating should be by an open grate. Gas stove heat is bad.

Out of Doors.—In the summer the baby may go outdoors when one week old; in the winter on warm, pleasant days when three months old. Keep the baby out of the wind. In windy, snowy or wet weather, do not take the baby out.

When the baby is a month old, except in cold and inclement weather, the windows of the nursery may be opened wide at times, all doors being shut to avoid drafts, and the baby thus given fresh air while dressed or in the crib.

He may be taken out in a carriage when eight months of age, and when the temperature is not below freezing.

To Prevent "Colds."—Never expose the baby to drafts or sudden chillings. Do not overdress indoors, and do not keep the nursery overheated. As the baby sits in the warm water, at the end of the daily bath, gently sponge the back and chest with cold water; but the temperature of the cold water should not be below 60° Fahrenheit.

Weight.—From birth until one week old, the baby will, in nearly every case, lose weight. For the first six months, there should be an average gain of from four to eight ounces a week, and from then to one year of age, from two to four ounces a week. The baby should weigh at three months about twelve pounds, at nine months about seven-

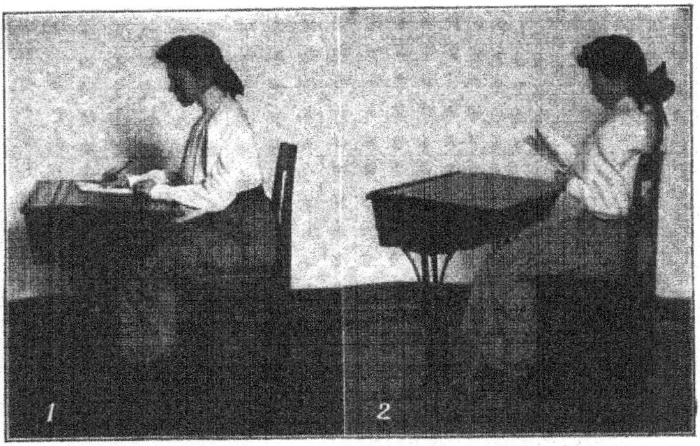

CORRECT POSITION FOR A CHILD AT A DESK AND STUDYING

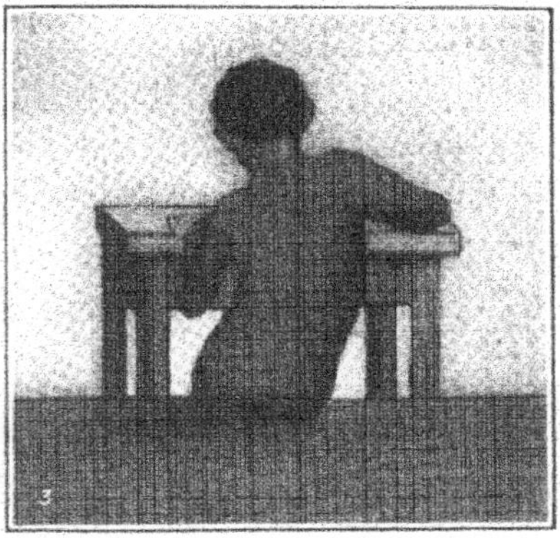

INCORRECT POSITION, SHOWING THE LATERAL CURVATURE OF THE SPINE RESULTING teen pounds, and at one year about twenty pounds.

Loss of weight usually indicates improper or insufficient feeding.

The Fontanelles or Open Spots in Skull.—The Fontanelles are the open spaces where the bones of the baby's skull do not quite meet. There are two—one kite-shaped, the other triangular.

At from fourteen to eighteen months these should be entirely closed. If there is any opening at the end of the second year, an arrested development is indicated and medical advice should be sought.

Facts Concerning the Baby.—A healthy baby should be able to hold up its head by the third or fourth month. It should sit unsupported, and crawl or creep from the fifth to the eighth month and stand when a year old. At about fifteen months it will try to walk unassisted. Do not permit this, as it is harmful and may cause deformities of the legs. Some babies of unusual strength walk when a year old or even sooner. It is best not to encourage precocity at this period of life.

When a year old, the baby will pronounce simple words, as "Mamma" or "Papa." If, at the age of two years it has not attempted to speak, see a doctor, as the fact will indicate an arrest of development, deafness or the first signs of idiocy.

There are exceptions to all these general rules.

Children usually shed no tears before the third or fourth month and the saliva appears likewise about the third month.

The healthy movement of an infant varies in color from a light orange yellow to a greenish yellow. The reaction is always acid. The smell should never be offensive, but should resemble that of sour milk.

The temperature at twenty-four hours after birth, is on an average 100.4° Fahrenheit; at forty-eight hours, about 98.6° Fahrenheit, and it varies little for the first few days. Later on, the average temperature is about 99° Fahrenheit. When a temperature is about 100° Fahrenheit, or below 97° Fahrenheit, something abnormal is to be expected. There is a fall of temperature normally in the evening amounting to one, two or even three degrees Fahrenheit. A baby's temperature must be taken by rectum, never by mouth.

The pulse varies from 110 to 150, consistently with health; it may be irregular consistently with health. When children are asleep, the pulse diminishes from fifteen to twenty pulsations.

Abundant perspiration is not observed in very young children.

A child should grow from six to seven inches the first year.

A new-born baby will sleep from twenty to twenty-two hours out of the twenty-four.

Do not get worried if a male child does not pass urine for the first day or two. This often happens. Always notify the doctor, however, so that he may make sure the fact is not due to any malformation.

Teething.—Teething commences usually from the fifth to the seventh month, and continues until the child is about two and a half years of age. The following table indicates in months the usual time of the appearance of teeth:

FIRST TEETH

Lower Lateral Incisors and 1st Molars	15 to 21 Months
Lower Central Incisors	6 to 9 Months
Upper Incisors	8 to 10 Months
Canine	16 to 20 Months
Second Molars	20 to 24 Months

SECOND TEETH

First Molars	6½ Years
Second Middle Incisors	7 Years
Second Lateral Incisors	8 Years
First Bicuspid	7 Years
Second Bicuspid	10 Years
Canines	11-12 Years
Second Molars	12-13 Years
Third Molars	17-21 Years

The lower jaw is usually a little in advance of the upper.

During teething the child's health requires unusual care, the bowels must be regulated, the diet strictly attended to and the gums carefully watched. The diarrhœa incident to teething is natural, and if in moderation should not be interfered with. A little castor oil is the remedy when the diarrhœa becomes griping, offensive or troublesome. Do not attribute all forms of restlessness and intestinal trouble to teething, but see a doctor, for there may be other and more serious conditions present.

Nursing the Baby.—In nursing the baby, note the following suggestions: If the mother massages her breasts and nipples daily for several weeks before the baby comes, she will find that her nipples keep smooth, the tender skin will not crack, and she will be saved a great deal of suffering.

After childbirth, wait for six or eight hours before putting the baby to the breast.

Put the baby to the breast every four hours until the milk comes, which is usually on the third or fourth day.

After this, nurse the baby every two hours, using both breasts, from 6 A. M. until 10 P. M., with one feeding at 2 A. M.

Do not nurse a baby more than twenty minutes at a time.

When nursing the left side, hold the baby on the right side with his head resting on the left arm of the mother, while the mother lies on her left side. The reverse is true when the baby nurses the other breast.

When the mother sits up to nurse the baby she should lean forward and depress the breast with the fingers of her free hand so as to keep the weight from pressing against the baby's nose.

Observe regularity in nursing.

Give the baby water from the first; at first, with a spoon several times a day; later, from a nursing bottle.

Weaning the Baby.—The time for weaning depends upon the condition of both the mother and the child. A baby that is not doing well may be weaned at six months or even earlier. If all conditions are normal, weaning should not take place before the eighth month and should not be completed before the baby is a year old. Avoid weaning the baby during the hot months.

If the baby is not weaned by the eleventh month, begin feeding from a spoon or cup. After a child is a year old it should be made to take nourishment from a spoon or cup.

Early Weaning.—Early weaning of the baby should not be permitted without a doctor's advice.

It is the habit of some mothers to shirk maternal responsibility, and instead of nursing the baby, to feed it from the bottle. If the mother is strong and healthy, with plenty of good milk, the baby cannot thrive on anything else so well. Many children are handicapped through life, invalids from childhood, because the mother shirked her duty.

In many cases, however, it becomes necessary for a mother to wean her baby before the usual time. Should a mother be tuberculous, it is better for the child to be fed by a bottle. This is also true should the mother have an infectious or contagious sickness, or should she be weak or suffering from any disease that is liable to extend over a protracted period. But in every case a physician should be consulted. The reasons for this are many:

He alone is competent to give a milk formula for the baby. Making up a milk mixture is not the simple thing many people imagine it to be. The age of the child, the physical conditions and the time of year—all are factors that a physician must consider. A formula that will suit one baby three months of age, another baby of the same age would starve on. One baby thrives on food which, if given to another, would cause intestinal troubles.

Patent Baby Foods.—There are many baby

foods on the market, advertised extensively, with testimonials "proving to you" the babies' lives it has saved.

Do not be deceived. Such advertisements are, for the most part, a delusion and a snare. Do not buy these foods and then feed the baby according to the directions. Your baby may get one of the diseases of malnutrition, a condition hard to overcome. The trained eye can detect grown-up people who suffered from the errors of nutrition when very young. If there is a patent food that will do your baby good, your physician will know that brand and advise it.

Some ignorant mothers think that condensed-milk-and-water is sufficient for the nourishment of the baby. The hospitals in all large cities have hundreds of babies entered on their records, little bits of skin and bones, and the history the mother gives is that her child was fed with condensed milk or with one of the popular brands of patent food.

From a financial standpoint, it will usually be cheaper, in the long run, to consult a physician, have him tell you the ingredients to use, and then make the mixture yourself, than to buy the ready-made foods.

Food Formulas.—At different ages the food percentages change. A child of six months requires different nourishment from one at two months. Many people begin to feed a child at one month of age, and, because the baby has done well, continue the same feeding. Then they wonder why the baby is thin and sickly and frets at five months of age. If in the beginning no mistakes are made the child will thrive and grow up healthy and vigorous.

It may happen that a mother will be suddenly prevented from nursing her baby and a physician cannot be consulted for several days. In this case the baby may be fed on the following formula until the doctor comes:

Let a quart of good milk stand six hours after it is received. Take off the upper nine ounces, measured by a graduated glass marked in ounces. If such a glass cannot be procured, a home-made measurement is eight teaspoonfuls to the ounce.

To these nine ounces, add two ounces of milk sugar, four ounces of lime-water and enough filtered water to make one quart.

The quantity given, should be two and a half ounces every two hours.

Let it be remembered that this is not for a continued feeding, but merely to tide over an emergency.

Care of Bottles and Nipples.—Any bottle, not too large, may be used to hold the baby's food. It is not the bottle, but the care of the bottle that is important.

Before filling a bottle, it should be boiled for ten minutes, or left to stand in water containing a half teaspoonful of baking soda.

Once a day, the bottles should be washed, both inside and out, with a bottle brush and soap and hot water.

Never refill a bottle that has not been properly cleansed.

The nipples should be allowed to soak in a solution of boric acid and water when not in use. Once a day they should be turned inside out and thoroughly washed with hot soap-suds. Two or three times a week they should be boiled for ten minutes. Put the nipple directly on the bottle. Do not use a contrivance in which the nipple is connected with the bottle by a tube.

OTHER FOODS PERMITTED THE FIRST YEAR

White of Egg.—Cooking the egg—Boil water in a pan and then drop in an egg. Allow the water to cool. After ten minutes remove the egg. Only the white of the egg is used. It may be given, beginning at six months of age; at first, one-half of the white of an egg daily, and at the end of a week the entire white of an egg may be used.

Beef Juice.—The juice should be squeezed from a lightly broiled steak. It may be given to a child about the eighth or ninth month. Give the beef juice before the milk feeding, and dilute it with an equal amount of water.

At first, only a teaspoonful of the juice should be given. Increase this amount every four days, until in two or three weeks two tablespoonfuls are given.

Orange Juice.—Only fresh juice, squeezed from an orange and strained, should be given. Give one teaspoonful at first, about an hour before it is time for the milk. Increase the quantity until four teaspoonfuls are given at a time. This should not be given until the child is about ten months of age.

Water.—It is necessary for the infant to have plenty of cool, fresh water, beginning at the time of its birth. Unless the water is known to be absolutely pure, it should be filtered before given to the baby. Keep it in a clean bottle for use. During the first twelve months, water may be given from a spoon, cup or nursing bottle between feedings.

After the baby is a year old about half a glass of water several times daily may be given.

Foods Given After Weaning the Baby.—Immediately after weaning the baby, nourishment may be given from a cup or a spoon. But until the child is eighteen months old, it is well to give it one bottle feeding a day, the morning being the time.

The foods may comprise milk, beef juice, mutton or chicken broth, a soft boiled egg and a piece of toast, fresh fruit, such as oranges or peaches, and cereals, such as oatmeal, hominy, farina or barley. Cook the oatmeal and hominy three hours. They may be given with milk, thin cream and a little sugar. Bread, at least two days old; also Graham crackers and scraped meat (slightly salted) may be given.

When the child is from two to three years of age bread and butter, toast or Graham crackers and a glass of warm milk may be allowed. Every other day the child may have a soft-boiled or a poached egg. The scraped meats should be either steak, chop, chicken, beef or lamb.

Among the vegetables permitted are potatoes, either mashed, baked or boiled; boiled rice or macaroni cooked soft with milk, green peas, spinach, string beans and celery. For dessert, the child may have either rice pudding, junket, custard, stewed prunes, baked apples, jellies or apple sauce.

For supper, it is best to give only a cereal and milk, or milk toast or bread and milk. A half a pint to a pint of milk may be taken at this meal.

CHAPTER XVI

HOME NURSING

Every woman at some time in her life has sickness in her family and most women have to do the nursing themselves. Few in any community can afford to employ a trained nurse. Volunteer nurses very often have more willingness and zeal than knowledge of how best to care for the sick and minister to their comfort.

The following are suggestions as to the proper methods of nursing:

How to Make a Bed.—The under sheet is first put on smoothly and fastened tightly at all four corners of the mattress. Next, a rubber protecting sheet is put on across the middle of the bed. Oilcloth may be used, if necessary, or even several thicknesses of newspaper. This protection is fastened tightly down at the sides of the bed. It is usually only as wide as a sheet folded double. Over the protector put the draw sheet. This is a sheet folded double and just covering the protector. If it becomes soiled, it is easy to draw it out from under the patient and to replace with another, without disturbing the protector or under sheet.

If the bed is for a person with a broken leg, the leaves of a table or a couple of ironing boards should be put under the mattress across from one side to the other. This gives a straight, unyielding surface on which the leg may rest without sagging.

If the bed is for a woman who is to be confined, make it as above, then add another protector and draw sheet. This top one is called a temporary bed and is to be removed after delivery, when the patient, with very little exertion, finds herself on a clean bed.

Moving a Patient.—No one should lift a helpless patient alone. Always have one helper. The nurse places one arm under the neck of the patient; this brings the head resting on her arm, her hand being passed under the arm on the other side; the other hand and arm are passed over the patient and under the middle of the back. The assistant passes one arm under the lower part of the back and the other under the knees, and both lift the patient at once.

To move a patient from one side of the bed to the other, the nurse places one hand and arm down the patient's back, thus supporting the head and shoulders, and passes her other hand over and slips it under the upper part of the back; the upper part of the patient's body may then be moved to the other side of the bed. The nurse's hands are then placed, one under the lower part of the back and the other under the knees, and the lower part of the body is lifted over. Another way is to loosen one side of the draw sheet, pull the patient over on that and then replace the sheet. To lift a patient off a bed, one person takes the sheet at the head and one at the feet. The sheet forms a sling in which the patient is carried safely.

BATHS

1. Foot Bath.—Get a small tub and have it ready with the hot water ordered, or the hot water and mustard. Loosen the bedclothes at the foot of the bed, and place over the lower sheet a piece of rubber or oilcloth on which to rest the tub. Place the patient's feet in the tub and pull the covers over all to protect from cold. Always dry the feet thoroughly after a foot-bath, and if they are cold apply a hot-water bag to them.

2. Sponge Bath.—Get the water and soap ready and have the clean clothes aired and at hand. Then remove the patient's clothes and wrap him in an old blanket. Only one part is exposed and bathed at a time. Begin with the face and neck, then the chest, abdomen, arms and back, and, lastly, the lower extremities. Change the basin of water at least twice.

An alcohol sponge bath is given the same way, only 60 per cent. alcohol is used and the parts are allowed to dry by themselves, while in the ordinary sponge the nurse dries each part as she finishes washing it.

3. Tub Bath.—When everything is ready the patient is either carried or assisted to the tub. He is then thoroughly soaped over, and the water poured over him several times from a large pitcher or pail.

In giving a cold tub bath for typhoid, one person must continually rub the patient all over to keep up the circulation, while the other pours the cold water on him and also rubs him. A hot drink is given before and after these cold baths, and the patient is wrapped directly in flannel.

HOT AND COLD PACKS

The Cold Pack is used to reduce temperature in many acute diseases.

The bed is first covered with a rubber sheet or oilcloth and over this a blanket. Then a sheet which has been wrung out in ice water, is placed over the blanket. The patient is laid on the sheet naked, and the sheet is wrapped around him so that every surface has the sheet next to it. The sheet is tucked in well at the neck and the feet. The blanket is then folded over the patient and tucked in. A wet towel is laid over the head. The pack should be continued ten or fifteen minutes. The patient is then dried and put back to bed.

The Hot Pack is given in a similar manner, only the patient is wrapped first in a blanket wrung out of boiling water. Two people, each taking an end of the blanket, wring it in opposite directions. More coverings are put over the patient than in a cold pack, and something cold is applied to the head, as an ice-bag.

FOMENTATIONS (*STUPES*)

1. A Hot-Water Stupe is prepared as follows: Take two or three pieces of old blanket and place in the middle of a towel. Then dip this in boiling water and wring out by twisting the ends of the towel in the opposite directions. Carry to the bedside and then shake the flannel out to let in air; it will then retain the heat much longer. Cover the fomentation with a dry towel and apply to the part of the patient for which it has been ordered. As this cools, have the next ready.

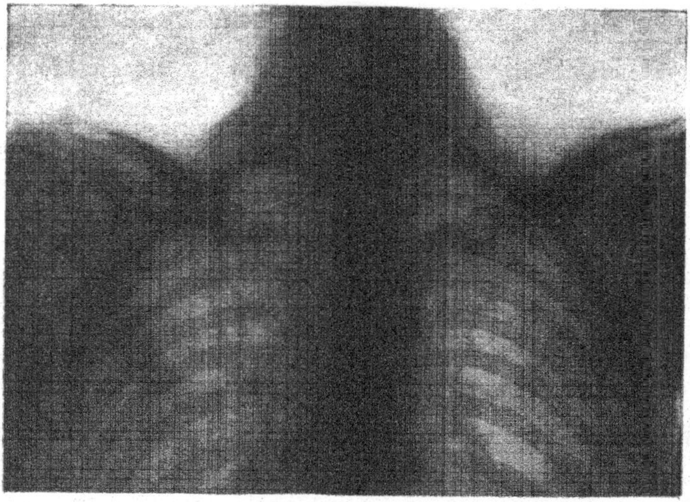

1. X-RAY PICTURE OF CHEST AND SHOULDERS

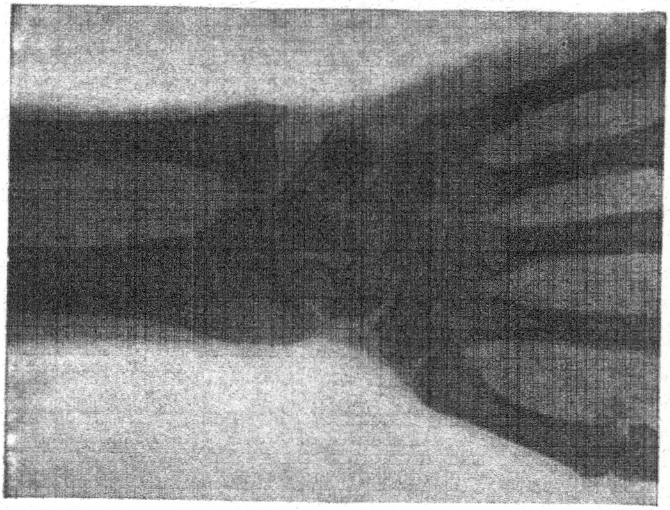

By permission of Waite & Bartlett Mfg. Co., N. Y.

2. X-RAY PICTURE OF THE WRIST SHOWING HALF A NEEDLE IMBEDDED IN THE WRIST

2. A Turpentine Stupe is prepared in the same way. After the flannel has been wrung out, sprinkle over it about thirty drops of turpentine, or to one pint of boiling water add three teaspoonfuls of turpentine and put the flannel in. Wring it out and apply as above.

3. A Mustard Stupe is made by wringing flannel out of hot water (not boiling) to one pint of which has been added one tablespoonful of mustard. Make a paste of the mustard before adding it to the hot water, to avoid forming lumps. Never use boiling water, as this destroys the action of the mustard.

Stupes are applied every few minutes, and when finally discontinued, the part should be dried and covered with cotton or flannel to prevent cold.

POULTICES

1. A Flaxseed Poultice is made by stirring the meal little by little into boiling water. When the mixture is like stiff mush, it is well beaten to remove the lumps. Then spread this paste, evenly and half an inch thick, on a piece of cotton or muslin, leaving one and a half inch margin for turning in. Cover the top similarly and apply to the surface ordered. A large poultice should be changed every four or five hours, but a small one every one or two hours. Do not remove until the new one is ready. Never reheat an old poultice; it is valueless.

2. **A Mustard Poultice** is made by adding two parts mustard and four parts of flaxseed to very hot unboiled water. The poultice is then prepared the same way.

Mustard Plaster.—A mustard plaster is made of equal parts of mustard and flour, or in the proportion of one of mustard to two of flour, one to three, or even, for very delicate skin, one to four. A paste is made with warm water, and this is spread between layers of muslin. It is applied and left for ten or fifteen minutes. When the skin is well reddened, remove the plaster.

Cantharis Blister (*Spanish Fly Blister*).—When actual blistering of the skin is desired, the cantharidal plaster may be bought, or cantharidal cerate (a paste) or cantharidal collodion. The plaster is cut the size and shape desired. If the cerate is used, apply it to some muslin first. Before painting with the collodion outline the part to be blistered with vaseline. This will prevent spreading.

It usually takes from four to six hours for a blister to form. The blister must be watched carefully, because in some people cantharides causes suppression of urine through its irritating action on the kidneys.

After the blister has risen, the lower part of it should be snipped with a clean pair of scissors. The skin is then allowed to heal over the spot of the blister.

ENEMAS

Definition.—An enema is a liquid preparation for injection into the rectum. It is given for various reasons: to relieve constipation, to check a diarrhœa, to give stimulants and nourishment and to relieve flatulence.

Enemas are either high or low. A high enema is an injection high up into the bowel. A rectal tube is usually inserted in the rectum, after being greased with vaseline, about eight inches. The patient is put on the left side with the legs drawn up slightly and the hips elevated, while the head and shoulders are low. A low enema is given with a rectal tube or a hard rubber tip to the fountain syringe.

Simple Enema.—This consists of warm water made soapy with any good soap. It is simply to evacuate the bowels, and is given high or low as the case may need. A protection of oilcloth or rubber sheeting is placed under the patient. The tube is oiled with vaseline or sweet oil;

also the nurse's first finger of her left hand is oiled. This is then passed to the rectum as a guide. The tube is inserted very gently upward and a little backward. The tube is held in place while the injection is slowly given. If given too rapidly it will be expelled instantly without result. If one enema is not expelled, in half an hour it is safe to give another.

Purgative Enemas.—1. Olive oil or castor oil. Warm six ounces of oil and inject as high as possible and slowly. This is to soften the movement. In about half an hour follow with an enema of one quart of warm soap-suds.

2. Glycerine Enema. Mix one-half an ounce to two ounces of glycerine with an equal amount of warm soap-suds and inject.

3. Turpentine Enema. Take one-half ounce of turpentine and mix with three ounces of warm water. In half an hour follow by an enema of soap-suds (about one pint). This is used also for flatulency (gas in the stomach).

4. Rochelle salts and Epsom salts. Mix one ounce of either salt and one ounce of turpentine with one pint of warm soap-suds. Inject high up.

5. Molasses. This is an excellent purgative. Take from two to ten ounces and mix with one pint of soap-suds.

Astringent Enemas.—These are given to check a diarrhœa. They are given very slowly, injected as high as possible, and the patient is encouraged to retain them as long as he can.

1. Starch and Laudanum. Boil the starch as if for the laundry and then dilute with luke warm water until it is thin enough to run through a tube. Of this take three ounces. This may be given alone in mild cases. Where there is great pain and tenesmus (desire to move the bowels and straining), and a doctor's permission has been given, add to the starch fifteen drops of laudanum or thirty drops of paregoric.

Stimulating Enemas.—Often in cases of shock, following an accident, after some one has been poisoned, or in the case of some exhausting sickness, it is necessary to stimulate through the rectum.

1. Salt Enema. Two teaspoonfuls of salt dissolved in one quart of hot water is mildly stimulating. To strengthen its effect, from one half an ounce to one ounce of whisky is sometimes added.

2. Black Coffee. Half a pint to one pint of strong coffee, strained before injection, and injected as hot as can be endured, is a powerful stimulant.

Nutritive Enemas.—In a few illnesses it is necessary to feed the patient by rectum. Of course, only a very limited variety of food may be given. Each enema should be preceded by a cleansing hot water enema, and then the nutritive enema should be given very high up in the intestine and very slowly. Such injections should never be given oftener than at four-hour intervals; otherwise the rectum will become so sore that they will have to be discontinued.

The most usual nutritive enema consists of: Peptonized milk, four ounces; white of one egg; a pinch of salt.

Beef juice, beef tea and other liquid foods have been given per rectum. If the enema is not retained, make it smaller until the bowel is accustomed to the process, or else add ten drops of laudanum or paregoric to the enema. This relieves the pain and makes the rectum tolerant.

DOUCHES

Definition.—A douche is a stream of water directed against a part, or used to flush a cavity, for purposes of cleanliness, or stimulation, or to relieve inflammation or hemorrhage. Three of the commonest douches are the aural, the vaginal, and the rectal.

Vaginal Douches.—A vaginal douche is given for

cleanliness and to relieve inflammation. For the former use only one to three quarts of water; for the latter use five to six quarts of water at a temperature of 110° Fahrenheit. This heat may be increased as the patient becomes accustomed to it.

A douche must always be taken lying down, with the hips raised on pillows and the knees drawn up. A bed-pan is put under the hips to catch the water returning. An ordinary fountain syringe with the long curved tip is used and refilled as often as necessary.

Aural Douche.—This is a douche of the ear. It is used in earache and inflammation of the ear. It is usually a hot salt solution or boric acid solution. It should be run into the ear gently and not with too great pressure.

Rectal Douche.—This is given to relieve the pain of piles and to reduce inflammation. It is given hot or cold, according to the doctor's orders. A rectal tube or a fountain syringe is used.

Antiseptic Douches.—The three most usual substances used are corrosive sublimate, carbolic acid and creolin. One tablet of corrosive sublimate to two quarts of water is strong enough. Carbolic acid and creolin must *never* be employed without the doctor's orders.

Use of Bed-Pan.—When inserting a bed-pan the

patient should be asked to raise the hips a little. The nurse then slips her hand under the back and inserts the flat end of the pan. This should be warmed previously by running hot water over it. Always raise the patient when removing the bed-pan; do not drag it out.

Disinfection (*Fumigation*).—Fumigation means the destruction of germs, usually by means of the fumes or vapor of some antiseptic substance.

All linen and clothes that are to be saved from an infected room should be thoroughly boiled. This will effectually destroy all germs. In the same way, dishes and silverware may be boiled and thus rendered safe.

A sick-room, after any contagious or infectious disease, should be thoroughly fumigated. First, everything that is to be destroyed should be burned, and everything possible should be washed in a 5 per cent. solution of carbolic acid. Sulphur is the best family fumigator. First, close all the cracks in the room at doors and windows by stuffing with cotton or pasting paper over them. All drawers and closets should be opened and pillows and mattresses exposed. A tub or large pan should be partly filled with water and two or three bricks placed in it, on which to put a smaller pan. In the smaller pan, put the roll sulphur, broken into small pieces and soaked in alcohol. After everything is ready light the alcohol, which, in turn, will ignite the sulphur. Then leave the room and seal up the door. The room is left for twenty-four hours and then opened and allowed to air for twenty-four hours more. After this the woodwork and everything possible should be washed in carbolic solution (5 per cent.), after which the room may be considered safe. At least ten pounds of sulphur should be used for an ordinary room.

Applying Dry Heat.—This is done by means of bottles or rubber bags filled with hot water or bricks or irons heated. These must all be well covered with some thick cloth to prevent burning the patient. The water in the bags must not be too hot; for an unconscious patient the bags must be moved every fifteen or twenty minutes, and the temperature should be between 110°-115° Fahrenheit. Severe burns may otherwise result. Expel the air before putting the stopper in a hot-water bag. This will make the bag lie flat.

Applying Cold.—Ice-bags are filled with small pieces of ice; they must be covered with a towel or other cloth to prevent freezing the skin underneath. As the ice melts the water must be poured off and the bag refilled. Expel the air from this bag as from the hot-water bag. When an ice-bag is applied to the head or spine, it is best to put a hot-water bag at the feet. This counteracts the depression to the circulation.

Keeping the Records of the Sick.—In a sickness of any length, the doctor is sure to want records of pulse, temperature and breathing. He will want a record of the daily movements of the bowels and urinations, and the hours when medicine and food are given.

The home nurse should have large sheets of paper ready for this purpose. At the head it is best to write the physician's orders as to medicines and diet. Below, make the heading "Day Report." Then, as each food or medicine is given, record the fact with the time.

If the doctor wishes the temperature taken once a day, do it in the morning and write it down. If three times a day, do it at eight, twelve and four o'clock and repeat at night the same way. At the time of taking the temperature take also the pulse and respiration.

A clinical thermometer is necessary in taking a temperature. One may be bought for a dollar, and if one does not know how to use and read it any drug-store clerk or doctor will give instruction. A baby, an unconscious patient and a delirious patient should always have a rectal temperature taken. Others are taken by the mouth.

Insert the bulb under the tongue and have the lips closed on the staff of the thermometer. Keep it in the mouth one to two minutes.

The pulse is taken at the wrist. On the thumb side of the wrist and on the inner or palmer surface is an artery, large enough to be felt easily. Rest the index or third finger lightly on this artery and with a watch in hand count the beats per minute.

Breathing is best counted when the patient does not know what the nurse is doing. Take hold of the patient's wrist as if to count his pulse, resting both his and your hand on his chest. Count the respirations in that position by feeling the rise and fall of the chest. One rising and one falling constitute a respiration.

General Care of Patient.—In nursing the sick, it is important to have the surroundings quiet and comfortable.

Do not speak of the case before the patient. Keep the chart containing the records of his illness in a place safe from him.

Visitors, if permitted, should remain only a few minutes at the most. Very sick patients should have absolutely no visitors.

Let nothing arise that may disturb the patient mentally. In governing a patient, always be tactful and gentle.

Kindness, a smiling face, little fuss, and the general air of optimism will do much to cheer a patient and start him on the road to good health.

APPENDIX

BATHS—1. Foot Bath.—(Best given in bed.) Small tub or basin used. Knees drawn up and feet put in tub. Bed clothes over all.

(a.) Hot water.

(b.) Mustard, a tablespoonful to gallon of hot water.

2. Sponge Bath.—Given in bed. Only the part being sponged is exposed. Each part dried and covered before proceeding to the next.

(a.) Warm water.

(b.) Cold water.

(c.) Alcohol and water: equal parts.

3. Tub Bath.—Patient is carried or assisted to bath, soaped all over and then water poured on him. If the bath is a cold one, the patient must be massaged vigorously during the immersion.

4. Turkish Bath.—

(a.) Dry heat room.

(b.) Soaping and massage.

(c.) Hot steam room.

(d.) Shower baths, hot to cold.

(e.) Cold plunge.

5. Russian Bath.—

(a.) Hot steam room.

(b.) Soaping and massage.

(c.) Shower, hot to cold.

(d.) Cold plunge.

BINDERS—1. Baby's Binder.—Made of flannel, four inches wide, with a three-inch lap over abdomen. Worn from birth until first year.

2. Obstetric Binder.—Made of any firm, strong cloth. Extends from chest to half way down the thighs. It is put on immediately after childbirth, drawn very tight and worn for ten days.

BLISTER—(*Spanish Fly, Cantharis*).—Caused by cantharidal plaster, cerate or collodion. Applied to area and left on four to six hours. After blister is formed, snip it with a clean scissors to let out the fluid.

CALAMINE LOTION.—Zinc oxide, one quarter ounce. Powdered calamine, one quarter ounce. Lime water, four ounces.

DIET.—1. Liquid consists of milk, albumen water, strained soups, orange juice, beef juice.

2. Soft consists of custards, junkets, soft-boiled eggs, milk toast, cooked fruits, cereals.

3. Full consists of regular table fare, excluding

such things as pork, corned beef, pastry, and other rich food.

DISINFECTANTS—1. Bichloride of Mercury, Corrosive Sublimate.—This is made in tablets which, dissolved in a pint of water, make a 1-1000 solution. 1-4000 is the usual strength used on the skin, although it may be used as strong as 1-1000.

2. Carbolic.—This comes in crystals or solution. Never use on skin stronger than 2 per cent. solution. For clothes or woodwork, use 5-10 per cent. solution.

3. Sulphur.—Soak in alcohol and burn in a room, previously sealed. At least ten pounds should be burnt in a room.

4. Formalin, Formaldehyde.—This is burnt in lamps which can be bought. Directions come with each lamp. Seal the room as in sulphur fumigation. This is a better method than the sulphur method.

DOSES—1. Amyl Nitrite.—Put up in glass "pearls." Break in a cloth and inhale fumes.

2. Calomel.—1 to 5 grains. Given in one-tenth or one-quarter grain doses every fifteen minutes, until the desired amount is given. Follow in six hours by salts.

3. Castor Oil.—One quarter to one ounce. Give in capsules or between layers of orange juice.

4. Compound Licorice Powder.—2 to 4 teaspoonfuls. Stir in cold water and give.

5. Compound Tincture of Benzoin.—One teaspoonful to a pint of boiling water. Inhale the hot steam, first making a hood of a blanket over both pitcher and the patient.

6. Fluid Extract of Cascara.—One-half to two teaspoonfuls. Dilute with water or essence of pepsin and drink.

7. Laudanum.—3 to 15 drops. Never give without a doctor's order. It is dangerous, containing opium.

8. Olive Oil.—May be given in any amount. Usually half a glassful is given at a time.

9. Oleoresin of Aspidium.—One-quarter to one teaspoonful. Given in milk, usually, on an empty stomach.

10. Quinine.—1 to 10 grains. Given best in capsules. Do not take in tablets or pills, as they are often not dissolved.

11. Spirits of Nitrous Ether.—Sweet spirits of nitre, one-half to two teaspoonfuls. Given in a little water.

DOUCHES—1. Aural.—Warm salt water, a teaspoonful to a pint. Run into the ear with not too much force. Boric acid solution, a teaspoonful to a pint, may also be used.

2. Rectal.—Given through a rectal tube or tip. Hot or cold water is used.

3. Vaginal.—For cleansing purposes plain hot water or salt water is used.

4. Antiseptic Douches are most used in the vagina. The following substances are used:

(a.) Bichloride of mercury, 1-4000.

(b.) Carbolic, a teaspoonful of a concentrated solution to a quart of water.

(c.) Creolin, teaspoonful to a quart of water.

ENEMAS—1. Simple Enema.—Made of warm soap-suds and water. Injected either high up in the rectum with a rectal tube or low in the rectum with the ordinary tip.

2. Purgative Enema.—(a.) One-half to two ounces of glycerin, in half pint of warm soap-suds.

(b.) One ounce of turpentine in half a pint of warm water. Follow in half an hour by a soap-suds enema.

(c.) Rochelle salts and Epsom salts, one ounce of each. Add one ounce of turpentine and one pint of soap-suds.

(d.) Olive oil or castor oil, six ounces of warm oil injected slowly.

(e.) Molasses, 2 to 10 ounces, added to one pint of soap-suds.

3. Astringent Enemas.—(a.) Boil starch as if

for the laundry. Dilute with warm water until very thin. Inject 3 to 5 ounces very slowly. Add thirty drops of paregoric or fifteen drops of laudanum, with a doctor's permission.

4. Stimulating Enema.—(a.) Salt enema. Add one teaspoonful to a pint of water. Inject about 1 to 2 pints slowly as hot as can be borne. Add 1 to 2 ounces of whisky in some cases.

(b.) One-half to one pint of strong hot black coffee, strained.

5. Nutritive Enemas.—Precede with cleansing enema of salt solution. Give high up and very slowly, at four to six-hour intervals.

(a.) Peptonized milk, four ounces. White of one egg. A pinch of salt.

(b.) Beef juice.

(c.) Other liquid foods.

FOOD FORMULA FOR BABIES.—Let one quart of milk stand six hours. Take the upper nine ounces of this. Add two ounces of milk sugar. Add four ounces of lime water. Add enough filtered water (unboiled) to make a quart. Feed baby every two hours, with two and a half ounces.

FOODS.—1. Egg Albumen.—Take the white of one raw, fresh egg. Mix it with a glass of cold water. Add a little orange juice or lemon juice and a pinch of sugar.

2. Beef Juice.—Slightly broil a small steak, and thoroughly squeeze out the juice. Add a little salt and give hot.

3. Salisbury Steak.—Take an ordinary steak. Chop it very fine and remove all fibrous and fatty portions. Broil, salt and serve hot.

FOMENTATIONS—(*See Stupes*).—

LAXATIVE WATERS.—Carlsbad water, Hunjadi Janos, Buffalo Lithia, Saratoga water.

These are to be taken before breakfast, 1 to 2 glasses.

LUNAR CAUSTIC.—This is silver nitrate in solid form. Used to burn any surface. The stick is wet with water and applied on the exact spot desired. Do not touch any other part, as it discolors and burns.

NOSE SPRAY.—Camphor, 20 grains. Menthol, 20 grains. Alboline, one ounce. Put in a vaporizer and spray the interior of the nose.

OINTMENTS..—1. Oil of wintergreen, two teaspoonfuls. Lanolin, one ounce. This is applied to rheumatic joints or rubbed on the back in lumbago.

2. Cocoa Butter.—

3. Vaseline, a mild, non-irritating ointment. Not absorbed.

4. Salicylic Acid Ointment, used in 5 to 10 per cent. strength for corns and calluses.

5. Nutgall Ointment, used in 5 to 10 per cent. strength for external application to piles.

6. Sulphur Ointment, used in 5 to 10 per cent. strength for scabies (the itch).

POWDERS—(*Dusting*).—1. Aristol.—An antiseptic powder used for wounds and raw surfaces.

2. Boric Acid.—Mild antiseptic powder.

3. Zinc Oxide Powder, a drying powder used in wounds and on skin to prevent chafing.

4. Zinc Stearate Powder, an oily powder used to prevent chafing and in some eczemas.

PLASTER—(*Mustard*).—Made of flour and mustard. Proportions vary from 1 to 1 to 4 to 1, according to the conditions. Make into a paste with lukewarm water, spread between layers of muslin and apply. Leave on until skin is well reddened or for twenty minutes.

POULTICES—1. Flaxseed Poultice.—Stir the flaxseed into boiling water until thick mush has been formed. Spread between muslin and apply. Change every two hours. Never re-heat an old poultice.

2. Mustard Poultice.—Add two parts of mustard and four parts of flaxseed to hot water which has not quite boiled. Apply as above.

SOLUTIONS—1. Baking Soda.—For a gargle or wash. One teaspoonful to a glass of water.

2. Bran Water.—Put a quantity of bran in a muslin bag and boil in water. Remove the bag after ten minutes' boiling.

3. Boric Acid Solution.—A saturated solution is used. Roughly speaking, this is a heaping teaspoonful to a glass of water.

4. Dobell's Solution.—May be purchased at any drug store without a prescription. Used as a nose spray and gargle.

5. Resorcin Solution.—This is a 2 per cent. alcoholic solution. Resorcin, 10 grains. Alcohol, one ounce.

6. Silver Nitrate Solution.—This is a 1 per cent. solution: Silver nitrate, 5 grains. Water, one ounce.

Used in inflammation of the eye. A drop at a time in the eye; then wash it out with boric acid solution.

STUPES—1. Hot Water.—Wring out flannel in very hot water. Apply.

2. Turpentine.—Do as above and then sprinkle on hot, wet flannel about thirty drops of turpentine; or add three teaspoonfuls of turpentine to a pint of boiling water. Wring the flannel out in it. Apply.

3. Mustard.—One tablespoonful of mustard to a pint of water, just coming to a boil.

Apply stupes every few minutes. When done, dry and cover part.

SALTS—1. Epsom Salts, one-quarter to one ounce.

2. Rochelle Salts, one-quarter to one ounce.

3. Citrate of Magnesia, one-half to one bottle.

Take salts on an empty stomach, preferably in the morning on arising.

WATER BAGS—1. Hot Water Bags.—Expel air before closing. Cover bag with towel. Never leave long enough in one place to burn the skin. For an unconscious patient do not have bags hotter than 115° Fahrenheit.

2. Ice Bags.—Fill with small pieces of ice. Expel air before closing. As the ice melts pour it off. Always protect from freezing by a thick cloth between the bag and the skin.

GLOSSARY

A

Abrasion: A break in the skin or mucous membrane.

Adenoid: A glandular tissue which grows in the back of the nose and throat.

Adhesion: Abnormal union of two surfaces as a result of an abrasion or inflammation.

Amyloid: Starch-like.

Anus: The extremity of the rectum; lower opening of the alimentary canal.

Aseptic: Free from contaminating or septic matter.

Asphyxia: The suspension of respiration and animation, due to the lack of oxygen in the blood.

B

Bright's Disease: An inflammation of the kidney, either acute or chronic.

Bronchiole: The small subdivision of a bronchus.

Bronchi: The two tubes into which the windpipe divides, called the right and left bronchus.

Buttocks: The fleshy part of the body posterior to the hip joints.

C

Cæcum: The blind pouch in which the large intestine begins.

Cancer: A malignant tumor; also called carcinoma.

Capillary: The smallest subdivision of a blood-vessel.

Carbon Dioxide: Carbonic acid gas. It forms part of the expired air.

Catarrh: An inflammation of the mucous membrane; especially of the respiratory tract.

Catheterize: To draw off the urine from the bladder by means of an instrument, called the catheter.

Chyle: The milk-white fluid formed during digestion.

Colic: A condition commonly called belly-ache; or severe griping pain in the bowels.

Collapse: Extreme depression or prostration from failure of nervous force.

Colon: The large intestine.

Coma: Unconsciousness.

Conjunctiva; The mucous membrane lining the eyelids and covering the anterior portion of the eyeball.

Conjunctivitis; An inflammation of the conjunctiva.

Constipation: Retention and hardness of the feces; costiveness.

Corrosive; A substance that destroys tissue, either by chemical means or by causing inflammation.

Crisis; The turning point in a disease or fever. A fever which falls by crisis is one that falls rapidly.

Cystitis; An inflammation of the bladder.

D

Delirium: A disturbance of the cerebral functions, characterized by hallucinations and delusions.

Dentition: The cutting or first appearance of the teeth.

Diagnosis; The distinguishing of a disease by its symptoms.

Disinfect; To destroy disease germs.

Douche: A stream of water directed against a part, or used to flush a cavity or part, of the body.

Duodenum: The first part of the small intestine, beginning at the stomach.

Dyspepsia: Impaired or imperfect digestion.

Dyspnoea: Difficult or labored breathing.

E

Ecchymosis: A leaking of the blood into the skin, due to an injury and causing a discoloration. Black and blue.

Edema; An effusion of serous fluid in the tissues under the skin.

Epistaxis; Nose bleed.

Eructation; Belching of gas.

Eruption: A skin symptom in certain diseases. Commonly called a rash.

Expiration: The act of expelling air from the lungs.

F

Feces: The excretions of the bowels.

Flatulence: A condition marked by the presence of gases in the alimentary canal.

Flatus: A term applied to gases in the stomach and bowels.

Flux: An abnormal flow of any of the excretions of the body; especially the feces.

Follicle: A very small cavity or sac.

Fontanelle: The membranous spaces of an infant's head, due to the delayed bone formation.

Fungus: A low order of plants.

Furuncle: A boil; a local inflammatory infection.

G

Gangrene: Mortification or death of a part of the body, due to failure of blood supply.

Germ: The simplest form of vegetable life. Some germs cause disease.

Glottis: The opening between the vocal chords.

Goitre: An enlargement of the thyroid gland. It generally accompanies cretinism.

Gonorrhoea: An infectious disease, usually of the genital organs.

Gripes: Severe cramps or colicky pains of the intestines.

H

Hemoptysis: The spitting of blood.

Hemorrhage: The flowing of blood from wounded or broken vessels.

Hygiene: The science which treats of the laws of health.

Hyperacidity: A condition of excessive acidity in the stomach secretions.

Hyperpyrexia: A condition marked by an excessively high temperature.

Hysteria: A functional disturbance or unbalance of the nervous system.

GLOSSARY

I

Ilium: The third part of the small intestine.

Immunity: The condition of the body wherein it resists the development of infectious or morbid processes.

Inspiration: The drawing in of the breath.

Intermittent: Occurring at intervals.

Intermittent Fever: Fever in which periods of normal temperature alternate with those of fever.

Irrigation: The application of water or other liquid in a stream to inflamed or abnormal tissue.

J

Jejum: The second part of the small intestine.

L

Labor: The process whereby the child is expelled from the mother's womb.

Laxative: An agent that loosens the contents of the bowels.

Leech: A small, worm-like animal, used in medicine to suck blood when applied to the skin.

Leucorrhoea: An ailment characterized by a muco-purulent discharge from the female genital canal.

Lumbago: Pain in the structures about the loins or small of the back.

Lysis: A slow decline of a fever to normal.

M

Malignant: A term used of diseases that increase with rapidity or that proceed to a fatal end.

Massage: Rubbing or kneading of the surface of the body.

Mastication: The process of chewing.

Menstruation: A monthly function of the female organism, evidenced by a bloody discharge from the vagina.

Microscope: An optical instrument for the magnification of substances too small to be seen with the naked eye.

Migraine: A sick headache.

Millimeter: (Metric System). A thousandth part of a meter. (Meter=39.37 inches).

Muco-Purulent: A term applied to a secretion of mucus mixed with pus.

Mucus: The viscid liquid secreted by the mucous membrane.

N

Navel: A round depressed scar in the middle of the abdomen, marking where the umbilical cord joined the child to the mother before birth.

Nephritis: Inflammation of the kidneys.

Neuralgia: A nerve pain.

Neurasthenia: Deficiency or exhaustion of nervous force.

Neurotic: Pertaining to the nerves.

O

Occlusion: A closing, blocking, or shutting up of a normally open aperture.

Oesophagus: The gullet. The canal leading from the mouth to the stomach.

Ointment: A salve or soft fatty mixture intended for application to the skin.

Opiate: Any preparation which induces sleep.

Oxygen: One of the elements constituting one-fifth of the atmosphere, and necessary for the life of animals.

P

Palpitation: Any spasmodic fluttering or tremor, especially of the heart.

Parenchyma: The essential tissue of an organ.

Pathological: Morbid or diseased.

Periosteum: A tough tissue covering the bones.

Pleura: The serous membrane which envelops the lungs and lines the inner surface of the chest.

Pregnancy: The condition of being with child.

Prepuce: Foreskin of the penis.

Prostration: Extreme exhaustion of nervous or muscular force.

Pruritus: Itching of the skin.

Puberty: The age when the young become capable of reproduction.

Puerperal: Petaining to the state of a woman in child-bed.

Purgative: A medicine producing watery movements of the bowels.

Purulent: Having the character of pus.

Pus: The fluid product of a suppurating wound, sore or abscess.

Pyelitis: Inflammation of the pelvis of the kidney.

R

Rash: An eruption of the skin, occurring in contagious diseases.

Rectum: The lower part of the large intestine connecting with the anus.

Reflex: A bounding back or return of an impulse.

Remittent: A term applied to any disease which has periods of increased and decreased fever. Between these periods the temperature does not reach normal.

Respiration: The breathing of air in and out by the lungs.

S

Sarcoma: A malignant growth; a tumor.

Scale: A small flake of detached skin.

Scar: A mark left after the healing of a wound.

Sedative: An agent that exerts a soothing effect on the mind.

Septic: Relating to putrefaction.

Serum: A yellowish fluid separating from the blood after the coagulation of the fibrin.

Shock: Depression of the vital centres.

Spasmodic: Pertaining to convulsions.

Sputum: A secretion ejected from the mouth in spitting.

Stimulant: A term employed to designate an agent for exciting the function of an organ.

Strain: An abnormal tension put on an organ or part.

Stricture: An abnormal narrowing or contraction of a canal or duct.

Stye: A boil of the hair-follicle of the eyelid.

Synovial Membrane: Membrane lining a joint cavity.

Syphilis: A constitutional, communicable disease, either acquired or inherited.

T

Tapeworm: An intestinal parasite.

Tonic: A medicine or agent which promotes nutrition and gives tone to the system.
Toxin; A poison produced from within the body or without.
Trachea; The windpipe.
Trauma: A wound or injury.
Traumatic: Pertaining to a wound or injury.
Tumor: An enlargement of a part; swelling; usually referring to a new growth.

U

Ulcer: An open wound that shows no tendency to heal.
Umbilical Cord: The cord-like formation through which the blood passes from the mother to the unborn child.
Ureter: The tube conveying the urine from the kidney to the bladder.
Urethra: The canal leading from the bladder to the surface of the body.
Urine: The secretion of the kidneys.

V

Vagina: One of the female organs of generation; a part of the birth-canal, situated anterior to the rectum; and extending from the womb to the surface of the body.

W

Wounds: A break or division of the soft parts of the body, caused by mechanical violence.

INDEX

INDEX

INDEX

INDEX

INDEX

Spotted something that isn't quite right?

Let us know and we'll fix it for future reprints. And as a thank you for your diligence, we'll send you a free Sothis book of your choice.

publisher@sothis.press

This page intentionally left blank

Made in the USA
Monee, IL
08 November 2026

67812160R00215